DYNAMIC CHIROPRACTIC TODAY

It is estimated that in Britain between half and three quarters of a million patients are treated by qualified chiropractors each year. In the United States, one in three Americans with back pain lasting two weeks or more consulted a chiropractor first.

Why? Because chiropractic gets positive results. The most thorough comparative trial of treatments for back pain yet conducted (reported on in the *British Medical Journal*, 2 June 1990) shows that chiropractic treatment is considerably more effective than treatment in National Health Service hospitals – so much more so that the medical researchers involved conclude that chiropractic should be included in the National Health Service.

DYNAMIC
CHIROPRACTIC
TODAY

The complete and
authoritative guide to this
major therapy

Michael Copland-Griffiths D.C.

THORSONS PUBLISHING GROUP

First published 1991 by Thorsons Publishing Group

British Library Cataloguing in Publication Data

Copland-Griffiths, Michael
Dynamic chiropractic today.
1. Medicine. Chiropractic
I. Title
615.534

ISBN 0 7225 1595 2

Published by Thorsons Publishers Limited, Wellingborough, Northamptonshire NN8 2RQ, England

Typeset by Burns & Smith Ltd., Derby

Printed in Great Britain by The Bath Press, Bath, Avon

CONTENTS

DEDICATION

This book is dedicated with affection and gratitude to the memory of Dr Glennys Foot, whose short working life embraced a quest for knowledge, a love of chiropractic, and devotion to her patients.

Born Ararat, Australia, 18 November 1946 – Died Aberdeen, Scotland, 3 December 1987.

ACKNOWLEDGEMENTS

In compiling such an all-embracing book on chiropractic I have had to rely heavily on the work of others, most of it absorbed over the years since I entered chiropractic college in 1973. The education I received at the Anglo-European College of Chiropractic implanted within me the desire to continue the search for knowledge beyond the excellent foundation it gave me, and I shall be forever grateful to those who taught me and fired my enthusiasm for my chosen profession.

In the mid 1970s attorney David Chapman-Smith ably represented the cause of chiropractic in New Zealand, since when he has devoted much of his time to researching and advancing chiropractic worldwide. His observations, published bimonthly in *The Chiropractic Report*, have provided me with invaluable source material and references, and I am grateful to David for allowing me to draw upon these.

Other non-chiropractic researchers have given me valuable insight into my profession through their published work. Historian Russell W. Gibbons, editor of the *Journal of Chiropractic History* and past president of the Association of Chiropractic History, has done much to identify and place into perspective the evolutionary stages taken by the chiropractic profession this century. Elizabeth Lomax's *Manipulative Therapy: A Historical Perspective from Ancient Times to the Modern Era* introduced me to concepts of 'spinal irritation' and helped me bridge the gap between old and new theories. Sociologist Walter I. Wardwell has contributed greatly through his numerous articles to my understanding of how chiropractic survived to become such a vigorous social phenomenon.

From within the chiropractic profession I have turned to many sources over the years. The *FACTS Bulletin*, published jointly by the Foundation for the Advancement of Chiropractic Tenets and Science and the International Chiropractors Association provides valuable statistics on the chiropractic profession and educational establishments worldwide, and gives a potted history of each national association. Much of my information on Australia has been gleaned from the work of Mary Ann Chance-Peters and Rolf E. Peters, editors of the *Journal of the Australian Chiropractors' Association*, and from the journal itself, and I am particularly grateful to them for checking and correcting the Australian sections of my initial manuscript as well as for their detailed criticism of the text. The Motion Palpation Institute's fortnightly newspaper *Dynamic Chiropractic* provides a regular round-up of major developments in chiropractic, often reporting on controversial issues that provoke heated argument from opposing viewpoints, and has been a useful source of worldwide chiropractic news. Its founder and first editor, Leonard J. Faye, took valuable time from the publication of his recent book on motion palpation to scan my first manuscript, and not only corrected a number of errors but gave several invaluable suggestions.

For anecdotes on the lives of Daniel and B.J. Palmer I turned to Vern Gielow's *Old Dad Chiro* and J.E. Maynard's *Healing Hands*, and these two works helped bring alive two of chiropractic's most colourful figures. Robert A. Leach's excellent book *The Chiropractic Theories* helped order my mind when tackling this massive subject, and he is probably the first person to draw together in one work the considerable advances of knowledge that have occurred since Homewood wrote *The Neurodynamics of the Vertebral Subluxation* in the 1960s. The results of Alan Breen's research in England have been widely published in medical and chiropractic literature and some of his statistics have been drawn upon. I am grateful to Alan for scanning my original manuscript and for his subsequent encouragement. George Walker, formerly Clinic Director at the Anglo-European College of Chiropractic, corrected several textual errors, gave me a number of very useful suggestions, and led me to several sources that I had overlooked. I am indebted to him for doing so in the midst of managing a very pressing examination schedule.

When it came to writing chapter five on the subject of exercises I turned to Sidney Hudson-Cook, a past faculty member of both Palmer College and the Anglo-European College, to review it. As a result I included a section on 'universal exercises', being a series of exercises that can be undertaken by most patients with the minimum of risk. His son Nicholas helped me integrate Sidney's suggestions into the manuscript.

Throughout the writing of this book, which spanned a period of three years, I have received encouragement from the British Chiropractic Association and from the Anglo-European College of Chiropractic. Principal Arne Christensen allowed me full use of the college facilities, making my job much easier. The college librarian has been particularly helpful in tracing obscure references, and use of the massive college library has proven invaluable. Students' Union President Keith Walker helped me find a model, Gesine Hoper, to learn and demonstrate the exercises. Tony Hunt photographed her, and Alison Marsh at Thorsons converted these photographs into line drawings. My secretary, Anne Payne, was an obedient 'patient' for the practical photographs.

Although I sought the advice of many colleagues when writing *Dynamic Chiropractic Today* I needed the insight of someone outside the profession to cast a critical eye over its form and contents. Peter Foot, Ph.D., as a true friend should, was not afraid to point out the shortcomings of my initial manuscript. As a result of his observations I was able to look at it under a new light, and set about restructuring and reordering the chapters to make it more readable.

Few publishing houses can have an editor-in-chief as tolerant as Thorsons' John Hardaker, and I am grateful to him for his patience when deadline after deadline was missed. With this first venture into print I had to turn to him on a number of occasions for advice, and appreciating my hectic daily schedule, he travelled to my home in Wiltshire to spend a day running through the penultimate manuscript.

The person to whom I owe the greatest debt of gratitude is my wife and closest friend, Penny. Always there at my side to organize my busy practice and social life, when these were being neglected day and night by my adhesion to a temperamental word processor, she not only fed and nurtured me but calmed my nerves when things went wrong. They often did. Without Penny's constant encouragement I am sure I would never have got beyond the first chapter.

PREFACE

There are a number of introductory books on chiropractic, but most are thumbnail sketches designed to whet the appetite. There are also booklets and pamphlets which guide the reader towards gaining and maintaining optimum health through diet, posture, exercise, and ergonomics. The chiropractic student will be exposed to lectures, books, and articles explaining the theory and practice of his or her chosen profession and to sources which help to place chiropractic in its historic context, but these are often couched in technical terms or are not readily available. There has yet to be an accessible book written to bring all these factors together in context, and this is what I aimed to achieve when I set out to write *Dynamic Chiropractic Today*.

In a mere ninety-five years chiropractic has grown from a tiny profession – outlawed and ridiculed – to become the third largest independent health profession in the Western world, after medicine and dentistry. This book reveals the background to chiropractic's remarkable achievements, uncovers its more shameful episodes, displays its dynamic strengths and exposes its weaknesses. It explains how chiropractic has thrived in spite of competition from other manipulative methods, and how chiropractic's distinct approach has set it apart as the pre-eminent force in international manipulative medicine.

The first five chapters are devoted to the potential patient. There must be tens of thousands of sufferers who live each day without relief, through fear of the unknown. By the end of this section you should feel familiar with what chiropractors treat, how they go about examining and treating the patient, what to expect after treatment, and what sort of follow-up is required. You will be guided through the care of your spine, helped through matters some might feel too shy to mention, told what to look out for if trouble is brewing, and given tips on what first-aid to apply if pain strikes. A series of case histories illustrates a chiropractor's typical daily workload and shows how its often amazing results make chiropractic one of the most satisfying occupations to be involved in. Hopefully all this will allay any of the worries those of you unfamiliar with chiropractic may have before embarking on treatment. Finally, there are a number of exercises that will help you speed recovery after chiropractic care, and avoid problems in the future.

For many of you this book will provide the first opportunity to learn the background of a profession which has brought relief to so many suffering people. The next section introduces the early manipulative techniques that were the forerunners of chiropractic, and describes the birth and early years of the profession. These were the years which endowed it with the dynamic impetus so essential for its survival, yet which also sowed the seeds of dissent that have surfaced from time to time throughout its history.

The development of the profession is mirrored by the development of its theoretical foundations from ideas which were in vogue during the nineteenth century to concepts of chiropractic founded on the latest scientific research. Chiropractic's philosophy has not been undermined by the scientific advances of the twentieth century but has been enriched and fortified by them.

Chiropractic is blessed with a massive range of manipulative techniques; originating with techniques that were designed to restore vertebral 'displacements', chiropractic methods now include those that best restore the dynamic function – or natural capacity for movement – which accompanies the healthy human frame.

The profession has more than doubled in size since 1977, and owes its modern outlook to a powerful emphasis on acquiring sound educational foundations. These enviable standards have been applied on an international scale, so that whether you seek chiropractic treatment in Stockholm or Sydney, London or Los Angeles, the quality of care you can expect from a qualified chiropractor is of the highest standard.

Because chiropractic has reached 'adulthood' in today's world of global communication and travel, it has been able to achieve its pre-eminent position in an organized manner. It has done so against massive medical hostility and propaganda, yet this has served to bind it together as a truly international movement. I have told the story of how this has been achieved on every continent, to give the reader an insight into the factors which have tempered this pioneering profession wherever it has settled.

The final chapter relates the position of modern chiropractic to medical and other professions, and gives an idea of how it will be fully integrated into the provision of health care during the next century. The coming years are likely to bring about great changes for all the professions that tend the sick and the suffering, and the dynamic nature of the chiropractic profession today will equip it to play a valuable role in the future.

I have attempted to keep all technical jargon to a minimum, and where chiropractic or medical terms do appear I have explained them. To avoid repetition or having to refer back through the text I have ended with a glossary, which has been considerably extended to act as a reference for further reading and to help you understand terms you might encounter from time to time in the future. Those of you who wish to learn will find a section on further reading, and there is another appendix with useful addresses.

Whether *Dynamic Chiropractic Today* is your first taste of chiropractic, or whether you have already experienced the benefits of chiropractic treatment, I hope that you will find reading this book an enjoyable and informative experience.

Michael C. Copland-Griffiths

Chapter 1

THE NATURE OF CHIROPRACTIC

It is most necessary to know the nature of the spine, what its natural purposes are, for such knowledge will be requisite for many diseases. *Hippocrates of Kos* (Fifth century BC)

CHIROPRACTIC: WHAT IT IS – WHAT IT DOES

The word 'chiropractic' is derived from classical Greek and means 'done by hand'. Chiropractors are specialist manipulative practitioners who concentrate on diagnosing and treating disorders of joints, muscles, bones, ligaments, and tendons. They usually pay particular attention to the spine, as its close relationship to the nervous system involves it in a great many cases of head, arm, trunk and leg pain, pins-and-needles, or numbness. Treatment aims to bring about an improvement or cure of many physical symptoms such as headache, facial pain, fibrositis, 'frozen shoulder', 'tennis-elbow', carpal tunnel syndrome, rib pains, lumbago, 'slipped disc', buttock, hip, or groin pain, sciatica, and knee or ankle pain.

The spine's close relationship to the autonomic nervous system, which controls all our unconscious functions, means that chiropractic manipulation will frequently help many other conditions seemingly not related to spinal disorders. Through the mediation of this autonomic nervous system, chiropractic corrective adjustment may help to banish or relieve such problems as migraines, vertigo, period pains, high blood pressure, water retention, constipation, bed-wetting, catarrh, and asthma.

CHIROPRACTIC FOR YOUNG AND OLD

Age is not a barrier to chiropractic care, and chiropractors treat both the youngest and oldest safely and effectively. Because chiropractors possess such a wide range of joint and tissue techniques they are able to select the most appropriate approach to the patient and the condition. With all patients, a full case history, physical examination, and diagnosis are made first. Most patients will be X-rayed to determine the state of their bones, to rule out any risk factors, and to help select the best type of adjustment – although in the case of children X-rays are only required in very unusual circumstances.

In very young children chiropractors will be on the lookout for birth trauma, or even injuries sustained prior to birth. The most common injuries to babies occur during a difficult labour, especially where forceps, vacuum extraction, induction, epidural or Caesarian procedures have been employed. Even traction on the neck during the later stages of a normal birth can cause problems. Not all spinal abnormalities are immediately noticeable to an untrained eye; chiropractors are often able to detect and correct these early problems, which might otherwise lead to such common conditions as migraine, asthma, or imperfections in symmetrical development, later in life.

As children grow through the crawling toddler and childhood stages, they will undoubtedly have numerous bumps, falls and jolts that can jar and stress the spine. Adolescence, often with difficult emotional stages and rapid growth spurt, can find children suffering postural stresses induced by depression, school furniture, or long hours in front of a television or computer. Contact sports during this stage tend to become more violent, and high insurance premiums reflect the greater incidence in young adults of road traffic accidents. Although a youthful body is better equipped to repair and adapt to injury, this factor frequently misleads us into thinking that all is well, masking abnormal movement that may surface decades later as 'spinal instability' and 'arthritis'.

Many of the problems found in adulthood and later life can be prevented or reduced by earlier chiropractic attention, but chiropractic can also ameliorate pain at later stages in life. Many conditions where patients are told 'You will just have to learn to live with it', can be helped by proper chiropractic care.

Arthritis, also termed osteoarthrosis or spondylosis, is one example of how chiropractic management can regularly bring relief, as the gentle mobilization of surrounding muscles and joints improves the movement of nearby structures, taking away strain from the painful area and bringing relief. Even though they cannot be cured, rheumatoid arthritis and ankylosing spondylitis can be eased with chiropractic treatment during their inactive phases, the chiropractor waiting for any inflammatory stages to pass before commencing treatment on the soft tissues closely related to the joint. Even degenerative conditions such as osteoporosis or osteomalacia can be relieved by a properly trained chiropractor and, as with arthritis, the pain of spontaneous vertebral fracture often found in the elderly can be alleviated by carefully increasing the mobility of surrounding areas, thereby allowing the painful joint to heal more rapidly, without any irritation from stiff joints that lie above or below it.

THE ROLE OF STRESS

A certain degree of stress is essential to healthy development; a seed must burst its case and force its way to the light before it can mature. A healthy body uses physical exercise to develop muscle, help pump blood and lymphatic fluids, and augment many body functions. Our mental capacities must also be stretched by solving problems to build up the basic blocks of our deductive faculties and form the foundation of the learning process. Likewise through life our emotional development is determined by the many hard social lessons we must learn in living with our fellow human beings. To develop in body, mind, and emotion we must undergo degrees of beneficial stress. Although extremes of stress will lead to breakdown, a total lack of it will lead to atrophy.

Extremes of physical stress may arise from accidents, faulty posture or technique at work, rest and play, poor mattresses, work-surfaces or seating, and weight overload, amongst many other things. Certain chemical elements such as tobacco smoke, car exhaust fumes, some foods and drinks, additives and pollutants are also unwanted stress factors when encountered in excess, and can damage health in one way or another. Psychologically, life may deal us cruel emotional blows that we are unable to adapt to or escape from. There are those who argue that cancer, and most other diseases, are stress related.

Stress overload of whatever kind may manifest itself in many different ways, but it always involves evoking the well-known 'fight or flight' response. The body physically tenses up in preparation for what, in primitive humans, would have been a physical attack or a dash for cover. The shoulders or buttocks tighten, the skull, neck and postural muscles tense up, and the abdomen contracts. When this physical manifestation is maintained for any length of time, existing physical problems will be exaggerated. Few of us escape life without at least some minor injury to our muscular and skeletal frame. Although healthy adaptation will drive away all the symptoms of these minor imperfections, the addition of undue and sustained stress of any kind upsets that adaptation by raising overall muscle tension. Increased structural malfunction occurs at our weakest spot, whether it be neck, middle, or lower back, and pain is felt locally or refers to the head, chest or limbs. A weak organ may itself start to malfunction, or a spinal problem may trigger an autonomic response that leads to disturbance of one or more of the organ systems. Frequently pain feeds back to overload the psychological system, creating a vicious circle. Many patients are told 'pull yourself together' by an insensitive doctor, who labels their unbalanced psychological state as the causative factor when it is merely a symptom. Chiropractors often become the last desperate port of call for patients who have been drugged by tranquillizers or else abandoned by an unforgiving system.

THE CHIROPRACTIC PRINCIPLE

Unlike medicine, which aims to identify, isolate, and then eradicate disease with a direct external force such as surgery or drugs, chiropractic's goal is to build up the body's natural resistance to disease from within. It presupposes that we all possess an innate force which resists disease, initiates repairs, and adapts alternative functions to maintain optimum health. Early chiropractors called this 'Innate Intelligence', whilst scientists labelled it homoeostasis. If the balance of this homoeostatic force is disturbed we are more likely to succumb to illness, are less able to recover from sickness or injury, and are badly equipped to develop compensatory mechanisms when tissue destruction has taken place. The chiropractor must examine the patient as a whole to determine why this innate force is failing to function properly; in this sense chiropractic is essentially holistic. However, education and training will have led the chiropractor to specialize primarily in restoring full function to the complex neuro-musculo-skeletal system which is central to good health. Although a practitioner may try to mediate a patient's emotional and spiritual condition, it is the patient's state of physical well-being which will be concentrated upon.

SPINAL FUNCTION

The spine possesses a number of functions. Not only is the central skeletal system the anchorage point for the arms, legs, and rib cage, but the twenty-four vertebrae that stretch between the base of the skull and the pelvic sacral bone allow an amazing degree of mobility as we bend forwards, backwards, sideways, and around. This flexibility, combined with our upright stance, has given us dominance over all other creatures in the animal

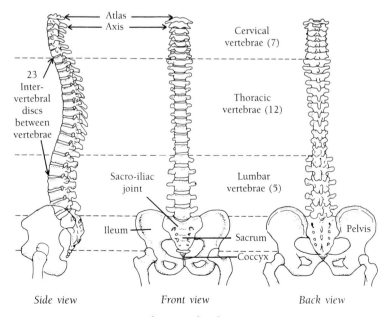

Atlas
Axis
Cervical vertebrae (7)
23 Inter-vertebral discs between vertebrae
Thoracic vertebrae (12)
Sacro-iliac joint
Lumbar vertebrae (5)
Ileum
Sacrum
Coccyx
Pelvis

Side view   Front view   Back view

The spinal column

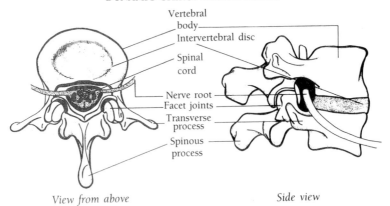

View from above   *Side view*

Basic anatomy of a vertebra

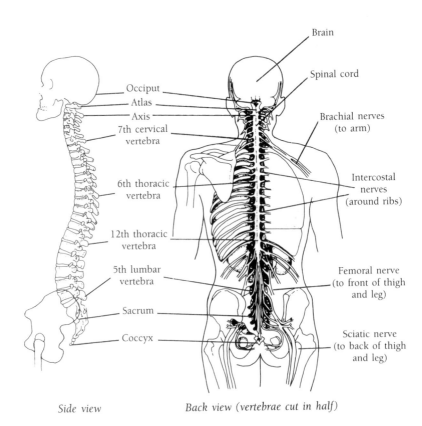

Side view   *Back view (vertebrae cut in half)*

View of the spine showing relationships of the spinal cord and nerves of the arm, leg and trunk

kingdom, enabling early humans to hunt for food, to flee from danger, and to thrive throughout the earthly domain.

This degree of speed and mobility requires a complex system of co-ordination and command which is provided through the central nervous system. Many functions, such as recoiling from a burn or maintaining bowel control, originate in the spinal cord; that age-old story of a farmer chasing a headless chicken, though fanciful, relies on the observation of movement under exclusive spinal control. All our actions and reactions are governed by the delicate nervous tissues that lie encased within our skull and vertebral column, so that the spine's other major role is a protective one.

To be totally protective the spinal casing would need to be solid and continuous, but this would sacrifice considerable mobility. In the human, therefore, there is an optimum balance between protection and mobility, with each compromise toward mobility increasing the risk of damage to spinal nervous tissues. Our flexibility leaves us vulnerable to nerve disorders ranging from mild tingling to total paralysis in the joints, muscles, and other tissues that make up our locomotor system.

THE AUTONOMIC NERVOUS SYSTEM

The autonomic nervous system controls our body functions automatically, without our conscious intervention. Our heart pumps blood, our lungs inhale and exhale air, our digestive system extracts energy from food and expels the waste, our kidneys maintain delicate chemical balances, our liver detoxifies us, our reproductive system creates and sustains new life, cells multiply, grow, die, and are replaced, and complex hormones, enzymes, and other body chemicals are manufactured and released, all without the need of our conscious intervention.

Because our body organs operate through the autonomic nervous system, and this in turn communicates with the central nervous system that lies encased by skull and vertebrae, disorders of the spine can at times upset the delicate controls that govern the cardiac, respiratory, reproductive, urinary, digestive, endocrine, and neurological systems. The chiropractor is therefore trained to detect and correct spinal disorders, but in

Connections of the autonomic nervous system showing schematic links between the brain, spinal cord, and body organs

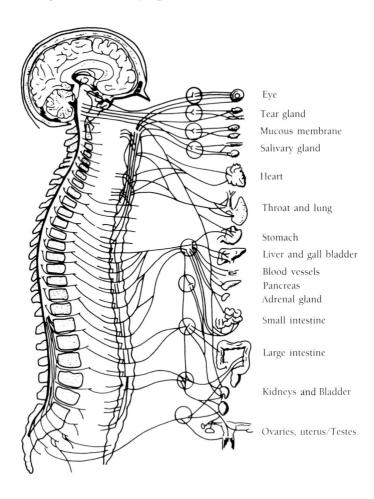

Eye
Tear gland
Mucous membrane
Salivary gland

Heart

Throat and lung

Stomach
Liver and gall bladder
Blood vessels
Pancreas
Adrenal gland
Small intestine

Large intestine

Kidneys and Bladder

Ovaries, uterus/Testes

doing so needs to be trained to differentiate these disorders from disease processes which are more appropriately treated by conventional or other forms of medicine.

THE CHIROPRACTIC SUBLUXATION

Chiropractors use the term subluxation to describe the spinal abnormalities they detect. The medical term luxation refers to joint dislocation, and the term subluxation originally described that state believed by founder D.D. Palmer and other pioneer chiropractors to be 'sub' – 'less than' – a full-blown dislocation. Because of the involvement of the nervous system the term took on autonomic and other neurologic implications. With a fuller understanding of spinal mechanics developing over the last forty years, the term is also used today to describe any abnormality of movement. Medical manipulators and osteopaths would tend to equate spinal subluxation with their own term spinal lesion.

QUALIFIED TO DIAGNOSE

Spinal pain does not always relate directly to disorders of the joints and may mask other underlying medical conditions. When consulting a chiropractor for any condition it is of paramount importance that you should consult one who is a fully qualified Doctor of Chiropractic (D.C.) with the minimum four-year full-time training that equips him or her to examine and diagnose other pathologies. The only other internationally recognized chiropractic qualifications are the B.Appl.Sc. (Chiro) granted to Australian graduates, and the B.Sc. Chiropractic degree to be awarded to British graduates from July 1991. Although useful, it is not enough to rely totally on a General Medical Practitioner for health screening, for qualified chiropractors frequently detect conditions requiring medical care that have been missed by the medical physician, either because no physical examination was performed, or through human error, or because the disease was then in an early, undetectable stage.

COMMONEST CONDITIONS

Probably more than 95 per cent of a chiropractor's patients seek treatment for bone, joint, muscle, or tendon pain in its many forms; included in this category are types of head pain related to tension at the base of the skull as well as referred arm and leg pains. Disorders primarily of the lower back and pelvis, including those referring to the groin, thigh, legs, feet or toes would account for about 50 per cent of cases. Neck problems causing local pain or referral to the shoulder, chest, arm, elbow, hand or fingers would account for about 25 per cent, and headaches and migraine for about 10 per cent. Thoracic pain reaching around the ribs or between the shoulder blades probably makes up around 8 per cent. Local injuries directly to limbs and not immediately involving the spine would account for about 5 per cent. The remaining 2 per cent of patients would be those whose spinal problems have manifested themselves not as musculo-skeletal conditions but predominantly as organic disorders acting through the autonomic nervous system. These figures are guidelines showing the predominant area of complaint, and take no account of the fact that very many patients arrive with combinations of head, neck, thoracic, or lumbar pain or with co-existing organic problems. Indeed, the majority of patients who secure relief from organic conditions arrive for treatment of a musculo-skeletal complaint, and it is only during the taking of case history that a possible autonomic involvement is revealed.

These figures would probably apply to most chiropractors worldwide, although in remote parts of North America and in some Third World countries the chiropractic physician in a rural setting may be the nearest physician. In these cases they may care for a family's health from cradle to grave, and some state legislatures permit chiropractors to deliver babies, conduct minor surgery, and sign death certificates. Indeed, the depth of a chiropractor's training in pathology, diagnosis, and in the basic sciences provide a foundation that makes chiropractic a safe, valid and valuable alternative.

Chapter 2

VISITING A CHIROPRACTOR

One of the first duties of the physician is to educate people not to take medicine. *Sir William Osler* (1849–1919)

A qualified chiropractor is trained to take a careful case history, building upon this with a physical examination, and ending with any other diagnostic tests such as X-ray, urine, or blood analysis. He or she will then consider the information gleaned and come up with a firm impression or diagnosis of what is wrong. This procedure is very necessary in helping the chiropractor to determine whether they are likely to be able to help the patient, or whether they should refer the patient for a more appropriate treatment, either back to a medical doctor, or on to an alternative medicine practitioner. If a chiropractor can help, the information obtained from the tests, and particularly from any X-rays, will influence the adjustment selected and the advice given.

THE CASE HISTORY

The chiropractor's receptionist will normally take a few personal details, such as name, date of birth, occupation, address, and medical practitioner's name before you are introduced to the chiropractor. The chiropractor will then question you about your problem, and will ask questions about any pain you may be experiencing. He or she will want to know its origin and location, the times of day or night when the pain is worse, those factors which provoke or ease it, any symptoms which may accompany it, and whether you have suffered before. Depending on your answers your chiropractor will pursue specific lines of questioning until a clear picture points to the most likely causes of the problem. Details will be asked of your general medical history, and here you should mention any health problems past or present, illnesses, accidents, and operations which, although they may appear irrelevant to your main problem, may have a direct or indirect bearing upon it. It is frequently found that after chiropractic treatment for spinal problems many apparently unrelated conditions such as constipation, menstrual difficulties, headaches, shortness of breath, will be alleviated or relieved altogether.

THE CHIROPRACTIC EXAMINATION

As a patient you will be asked to change down to your underclothes, and women will be given a gown that opens down the back to reveal the spine. It is usual for your chiropractor to observe your spine for any obvious curves, signs of muscle

Motion palpation of neck

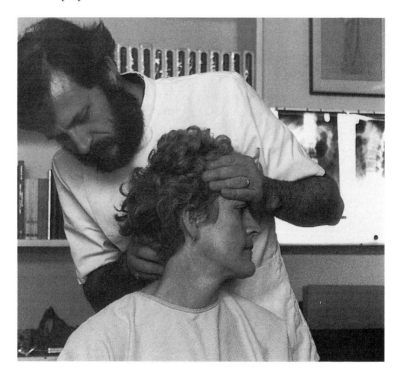

tension, and for general postural information. Patterns of skin colouring or glistening will be noted, as will surface temperature differences, since these are factors that can indicate any autonomic nervous system activity accompanying a subluxation (joint disturbance). Even a small tuft of hair at the base of the spine may offer a hint that below the surface the spinal bones have not fully formed, or are abnormally shaped. Your chiropractor may wish to observe you standing, sitting, walking, or lying down before moving on to palpate (feel) the spinal joints and tissues that surround them.

Palpation, or analysis by touch, involves judging the feel and texture of the tissue and normally follows the initial observation stage. Skin, muscle, ligament, and bone are all assessed and abnormalities noted. The chiropractor will then take you through a range of movements to determine which joints are performing normally, which are moving too much, and which are not moving enough. A joint may move perfectly well in one

Motion palpation of the low back

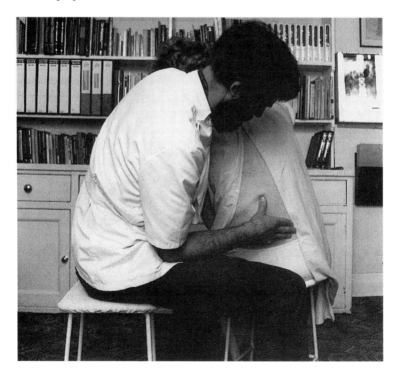

direction but not in another, so 'motion palpation' can involve a series of small manoeuvres around one specific joint, to determine whether bending forwards or backwards, from side to side, or twisting round one way or the other reveals a movement malfunction of that joint. In addition to faulty joint mobility the chiropractor may decide to perform certain muscle tests to determine strength and weakness under various circumstances, or may directly palpate one of the important postural muscles such as the psoas muscle, reached by pressing down by the side of the abdomen, or the piriformis muscle, which runs from the base of the spine to the hip joint.

Usually palpation will not restrict itself to the area of complaint. Any postural distortion will affect the whole body's balancing mechanism, and therefore has to be met by a counter distortion elsewhere in the spine or pelvis. The level of the eyes will remain constant to help us balance, so that if a damaged foot causes us to lean away from the painful side, this postural distortion will be compensated by the body leaning towards it somewhere else. Usually this takes place with a series of small curves and counter-curves, as the body overcompensates in the pelvis and in the spine, with a final balancing often taking place in the upper three neck vertebrae or base of the skull. Counterbalancing may also occur below the problem, so that a neck injury may elevate one shoulder and cause a side-sway, perhaps in the pelvis. Such compensatory distortions may themselves become restricted or over-mobile, and this is why your chiropractor may not just restrict an assessment to the area you complain about. He or she may choose to examine and later treat your muscular and skeletal frame at any point from the tip of your toes to the top of your head, even palpating the minute movements of the skull bones that accompany breathing, if it is felt they may be involved in your problem.

THE ORTHOPAEDIC AND NEUROLOGIC EXAMINATION

In addition to building up a mechanical picture of how the body is working from a chiropractic point of view, your chiropractor will want to perform certain tests that any orthopaedic consultant in a hospital would perform. One common test, usually conducted in cases of leg pain, is the straight leg raise, which draws the sciatic nerve roots through their spinal openings. Any pressure on a nerve root prevents it from being drawn through and leg pain restricts the leg raise. The femoral nerve roots may be tested in a similar way, as the knee is bent and the heel moved towards the buttock. Knee pain frequently has nothing to do with the knee and all to do with the hip, so a specific orthopaedic test for hip restriction or arthritis involves the thigh being drawn upwards and outwards to assess hip movement.

Arm pain is assessed with a series of arm and neck manoeuvres which challenge the pathway of the nerves as they leave the neck and travel under the shoulder to run down the arm. This outlet is composed of bones such as the upper ribs or collar bone (and in some cases a fibrous cervical rib from the lower neck) as well as several sets of muscles which anchor the head and neck to the bones of the torso. Abnormalities of these bones or muscles can cause arm pain. The wrist may also be tested to determine whether a thickening of the carpal tunnel (where tendons and nerves travel through to the hand) is causing pressure to the nerve and sensitizing it. Even in cases of true carpal tunnel syndrome, correct careful adjustment of a neck restriction will frequently alleviate such arm pain, as it appears to take the pain threshold of the nerve to a point where minor carpal tunnel pressure is no longer felt. Orthopaedic tests for the shoulder will be conducted where restriction is suspected, and will not only assess the full range of joint movements, but any painful arcs which occur as muscles and tendons are drawn by movement over hard bony surfaces.

Neurologic testing will include an assessment of the deep tendon reflexes, as these test the ability of the nervous system to sense the rubber hammer and respond with muscle contraction. Any interference along the sensory pathway to the spinal cord, within the cord itself, or along the motor pathway out of it may affect the reflex, and so a disc bulge onto the nerve root may sometimes alter it. As each tested reflex on the arms or legs is controlled by different nerve pathways, it is sometimes possible to diagnose the spinal level at which the interference occurs.

Further information may come from strength or tape measure tests on specific muscles, as these contract in response to impulses passed through the spinal nerves, and weakness or muscle withering may indicate the exact level at fault. Likewise the skin surface has nerve endings to record sensation and it can be mapped out to specific spinal sources of supply. Oversensitivity or numbness may be detected by pinprick tests which do not puncture but run lightly over the skin to reveal the exact point where altered sensitivity occurs, so the spinal level can be identified even though some degree of overlap with its neighbour exists.

In addition to testing the spinal nerves there are other tests for the twelve cranial nerves which may be applied by your chiropractor. He or she may also want to check your balance with your eyes closed, ask you to walk on the spot, ask you to cough hard, check your ability to sense vibration or temperature, or scrape the sole of your foot for a reaction. These and many other neurologic and orthopaedic tests may be selected according to your problem, and will help your chiropractor to build up a picture of the various parts of your neuro-musculoskeletal system.

MEDICAL SIGNS

Your chiropractor will want to rule out any medical factors that could be causing or complicating your condition. It is quite common for the blood pressure to be taken, the heart and lungs listened to, the blood-vessels behind the pupil of the eye looked at, and the ear and eardrum examined. Qualified chiropractors are trained to palpate the abdomen, to examine the breasts, to perform a routine gynaecological examination, and to palpate the prostate gland. In some countries chiropractors prefer to refer their patients to a medical practitioner for the more intimate examinations, and others will always leave this option open for the patient to decide. Nevertheless chiropractors have been trained to be on the lookout for problems or complications in patients that are best referred to medical practitioners or specialists. For example, headaches may relate not to the neck but to high blood pressure; jaw, arm, or chest pain to a heart problem; right shoulder pain to the gall-bladder; thoracic pain to a hiatus hernia; low back pain to kidney, uterus, testicular, or prostate problems; and leg pain to disturbances of circulation. These are but a few of the complications that your chiropractor has been trained to rule out before completing the diagnosis.

X-RAY STUDIES

Chiropractors the world over are trained to take X-rays, not only to rule out bone diseases that might mean referring the patient to a medical doctor, but to clinch a diagnosis and help determine the most appropriate form of adjustment. Chiropractors have been concerned for decades about the common hospital practice of multiple X-ray exposures, and they restrict the number of X-rays taken of an area to a bare minimum whenever possible, and follow the strictest codes of safety.

It is very common to find the presence of degenerative forms of arthritis on an X-ray, but chiropractic is at an advantage in that the X-ray will reveal the degree of damage and will help determine the best chiropractic approach. Earlier stages may indicate that conventional forms of adjustment can be safely used, but more advanced forms of arthritis may call for a non-force technique such as an Activator, or a soft tissue treatment like the Nimmo Receptor Tonus method. There are literally hundreds of options open to a qualified chiropractor, and the X-ray will help select the area of contact and the direction and depth of the adjustment.

Other common factors revealed by X-ray are irregularly formed joints, the absence of joints, and the existence of joints where none normally exist. A vertebra may sometimes become deformed and elongated so that the main body of the bone slides forward whilst the projecting part of the spine and small posterior joints remain *in situ*. A number of such common deformities or abnormalities may rule out the popular practice of low-back side-twisting manipulation or neck rotation adjustment, for these techniques sometimes induce painful reactions when applied without the benefit of radiographic information.

LABORATORY STUDIES

During training the chiropractor learns basic laboratory procedures such as urine analysis, and venipuncture to test the blood. These techniques help to rule out kidney, liver, or pancreatic malfunction from a specimen of urine, and blood samples can identify various forms of anaemia, abnormal blood cells, blood counts, or sedimentation rate, and incorrect levels of enzymes, hormones, or other substances that can indicate underlying disease. Your chiropractor may take and examine samples in his or her own clinic, but frequently sends blood samples away for laboratory analysis or refers you to your medical doctor for the tests.

THE DIAGNOSIS

When the case history has been taken, the chiropractic orthopaedic and neurologic examination performed, the X-rays read, and the results of any laboratory studies considered, the chiropractor will normally review these findings with you and may explain your X-rays. You will probably be told how the condition evolved, what has occurred to your muscles and joints to bring on the symptoms, and whether a course of chiropractic treatment is likely to be helpful. Some chiropractors will, with your permission, write a courtesy letter to your medical doctor either as a brief note or giving a report of the relevant findings and diagnosis.

THE TREATMENT

There is a popular misconception that chiropractic manipulation is a particularly vigorous procedure; in fact very little physical strength is required to deliver the chiropractic adjustment. Women should not be deterred from becoming chiropractors by imagining huge strength is required! Although there were fewer women chiropractors in the pioneer years, this applied throughout all the professions at that time, and in England more than 40 per cent of undergraduates at the Anglo-European College of Chiropractic are now women.

Once your chiropractor has completed the examination and made the diagnosis, there will be enough information available to select the treatment that best suits your condition. The adjustment may involve positioning you on a special treatment couch or chair that minimizes any discomfort, or you may be seated on a stool, or asked to kneel or stand.

If the chiropractor is to give a direct adjustment you will need to relax totally to allow the joint to be moved passively to its range of ordinary movement, known as the elastic barrier of resistance. When this is reached a rapid but very shallow

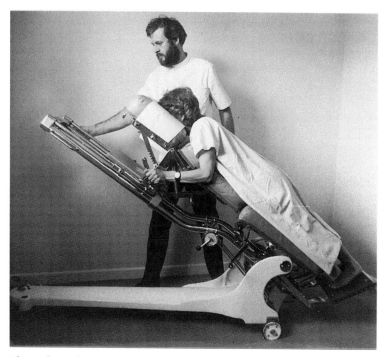

The Hilo – the most popular chiropractic treatment couch for more than fifty years

movement takes place, carrying the joint over this elastic barrier, but not so far as to stretch it beyond its full range of movement. This is the adjustment, and it is sometimes, but not always, accompanied by a click from the joint. The click occurs in a fraction of a second as nitrogenous gases are drawn from the joint fluid to coalesce as a bubble which then bursts with a 'pop'. Although this sounds quite dramatic the adjustment is normally quite painless. If pain is felt it is generally from the firm pressure over nearby inflamed tissues, not often from the adjustment itself, and normally clears rapidly.

If the chiropractor is to use that adjustment termed a toggle recoil, extra time will be taken in positioning you to ensure that the skin is stretched by the wrist placed firmly over the joint so it cannot roll off the precise spot. There follows a split second thrust as the joint is moved, but there is rarely a joint crack. It is the rapid speed of the adjustment and the recoiling away of the contact hand that creates a wave of relaxation around the restraining tissues of the joint, allowing it to return to its normal mobility and function, and inducing the neurological effects of the adjustment.

Some chiropractors may use an Activator or other instrument to deliver their adjustment, which is also very rapid, very measured, and quite painless. You may be positioned on a drop table so that one of its sections can be set to give way, dropping about an inch as a pre-measured force is reached, potentiating the effect of the adjustment and minimizing discomfort. Many chiropractors use such a table in conjunction with a toggle recoil adjustment.

Sometimes the chiropractor will choose an indirect adjustment or a non-force technique. You may be placed over a pair of irregularly positioned wedges or blocks which allow the force of gravity to make the adjustment. Light pressure may be applied while you breathe rhythmically, reflex points may be stimulated to influence blood or lymphatic flow, cranial bones may be eased, or muscles may be pressured, stretched, or massaged.

A number of chiropractors will occasionally use non-manipulative techniques when these are appropriate or when joint inflammation precludes a manual approach. Hot or cold packs may be applied, you may be given forms of physical therapy such as ultrasound, short-wave diathermy, and inter-ferential therapy, or strapping and tape may be used to stabilize a joint. Supports for joints of the upper and lower limbs may be prescribed, as occasionally are soft belts, corsets, or collars for pelvic or spinal joints. If you have a significantly short leg, or are developing hip arthritis, you may be given a cork wedge to place under your heel, or directions may be given for adapting your shoes.

There are times when specific exercises are needed, either to help you over a particular crisis or to act as a preventive measure, and your chiropractor will advise you on these. You should ask him or her to endorse any exercises you may already be doing, or which have been given by a friend, neighbour, doctor, or other therapist. You may have exactly the same symptoms as your neighbour or the last patient but the cause may be quite different; where one set of exercises may help one patient, they may not be appropriate for the next.

Your chiropractor may have asked you about your family life, occupation, or life-style if there are indications that mental, occupational, or dietary stresses may be involved. You should feel free to tell your chiropractor everything, as the Hippocratic

Oath they have taken together with the professional code of ethics ensure total discretion. Stress can play a major role in the onset of muscle or joint aches and pains, and there are times when we are unable to escape from stressful circumstances. However, chiropractic treatment combined with advice on posture, relaxation, exercise, and even on household furniture or work-surface design can reduce the overall tension levels considerably, enabling us to cope more efficiently with those stresses we are unable to avoid. As we start to feel better so we feel stronger, and management of our problems becomes better and better day by day.

Some types of stress can be corrected by altering our life-style. Such stress may be due to insulting the lungs with cigarette or cigar smoke, the digestion with junk foods or irregular meals, or physical well-being with lack of sleep, overwork, too much alcohol, or overeating. Some patients suffer sensitivity to certain foods, some of the commonest being refined sugars and flour, dairy products, coffee or tea, alcohol, and food additives. Others may be over-sensitive to chemicals in their environment such as components in paints, carpets, building and insulating materials, and cleaning agents. If these stresses can be identified and eliminated they reduce the body's overall sensitivity to other forms of stress and help overcome muscle and joint aches and pains.

THE FOLLOW-UP

Most problems have been built up over a period of time, usually with no apparent symptoms, so that one small movement such as sneezing, tying a shoelace, or turning in bed can trigger the first acute attack of pain. Often one or more joints have quietly seized up so that joints above or below have to compensate with extra movement. The ligaments that prevent a joint overreaching itself are slowly and imperceptibly stretched to allow for this, and a final twist or pull overcomes remaining stability in the joint, tearing or damaging its soft tissues. Muscle spasm then enters the picture, as nature supplies its own natural splint to prevent further damage to the joint.

Such damage cannot be put 'back into place' with one click. The adjustment is directed to the original seized-up joints, freeing them to take the strain off the damaged area. Often the restraining ligaments around the lazy joints have shortened, as they have not been subjected to recent use. Adjustment often has to be repeated on several occasions to restore a full and lasting mobility, and even when all symptoms have gone it is wise to have the joints checked once or twice more to ensure that they remain freely mobile and are not quietly and painlessly stiffening as a prelude to another attack. In some recurrent conditions, or where your job or life-style puts your back at risk, it is wise to visit your chiropractor periodically for a check-up, and your chiropractor will advise you how frequently you should be checked if you fit into a risk category.

Your chiropractor will want to follow up your first treatment soon after, perhaps daily or several times in the first week. They will warn you of reactions, for it is fairly common for increased joint soreness to occur after the first one or two treatments and this may last from a few hours to a couple of days. General muscular aches and pains may come on soon after treatment or several days after, and these may last from a few hours to a week. They are generally due to the stretching of ligaments and muscles that have previously been under-used, so now that locked joints have begun to move again their associated soft tissues are sensing unaccustomed use. Such reactions should give little concern as they are usually heralding a successful response.

Occasionally an earlier problem may rear its head as the presenting symptoms start to subside. This process, known as retracing, represents the reversal of your condition through its various stages. For example, a neck condition may bring acute pain which abates when the body develops a compensatory curve lower down in the spine to counterbalance and alleviate the original neck pain. Weeks, months, or even years later the compensatory low-back curve may induce an attack of acute local pain. This pain may then be treated with adjustment low in the spine that should be accompanied by treatment of the original neck condition if the problem is not to recur. It may not always be appropriate to treat both ends of the spine at once, or the low back may respond immediately whilst the more long-standing neck condition may take more time. On some occasions when the lower back is corrected it ceases to compensate for the earlier neck condition, and reawakens the old problem. This applies to any of the postural joints so, for example, an old low-back problem may become apparent as the neck is corrected, or headaches may recur when a knee or ankle is put right. You must be patient until all the postural elements of a long-standing condition are identified, treated, cleared, and followed up.

The follow-up period varies considerably from patient to patient and from condition to condition. Some patients may need only two or three treatments in total, whilst others may need a dozen or more. A survey conducted in Britain indicated that a patient receives an average of six to seven treatments before being discharged, and a recent American study put the majority of patients in a band of between one to ten visits. Generally speaking, a recent acute problem will rapidly respond whilst long-standing chronic conditions take longer. Some of the very long-term problems may be accompanied by irreversible changes, so that chiropractic treatment may only bring temporary relief, and a maintenance treatment is required every few weeks or months to prevent or lessen further deterioration.

Chapter 3

CHIROPRACTIC CASE HISTORIES

The most wonderful study of mankind is man. Relieving human suffering and diffusing universal knowledge is humanitarian. *Daniel D. Palmer* (1845–1913)

This chapter serves to demonstrate many of the typical conditions and experiences of patients under chiropractic care. Sample case histories have been given, but naturally a patient's name, circumstances, and sometimes sex have been changed to respect confidentiality, and some cases have been abridged or adapted for better illustration.

LOW BACK PROBLEMS

ALISON suffered constant low-back and leg pain for more than seven years following a gardening strain to her back. Her medical physician had prescribed heat, traction, exercises, a corset, and eventually surgery to a disc, but to no avail. She could no longer stand at an ironing board, sink, or cooker and for two years had been unable to carry shopping. Sexual intercourse was painful and this helped place burdens on a difficult marriage, so that when she sought chiropractic treatment she had been divorced for several months. Fortunately her teenage daughter stayed with her, was able to do much of the housework, and took her shopping in a wheelchair on Saturdays. At 36 Alison felt useless, rejected, and utterly depressed, so that few of her old friends or acquaintances had time for her any more. One friend, however, had benefited from chiropractic treatment, and insisted on taking her to see her own chiropractor.

The chiropractor diagnosed a problem with the fifth lumbar

disc but found that the right sacro-iliac joint (part of the pelvis) had not moved fully for years. Previous efforts to help Alison had been directed at the faulty disc, but no one had recognized the preceding pelvic condition that had overloaded the disc in the first place.

The initial treatment left Alison feeling sore and disillusioned for two days, and there was no reduction of pain until after the fourth treatment, ten days later. Now she started to improve, and within three weeks Alison was shopping on her own again. Five months later she met a new man, and they now have a nine-year-old son of their own. Alison enjoys playing with her young grandchild, and apart from the occasional twinge she leads a normal pain-free life. She visits her chiropractor twice a year to ensure that the sacro-iliac joint remains free, and still does a daily stretching exercise to help keep it mobile.

GEOFF has his own business driving a lorry, and contracts himself out to a local stone quarry. He had recently purchased a new vehicle on credit, and his heavily mortgaged house was his only security. To maintain payments on both he worked every available hour, and as he was paid for each load he never took things easily. Early one morning he slipped on the footplate and fell heavily on his right hip. Feeling little discomfort at first, Geoff carried on working, but as the day progressed he felt his back stiffen up. That night he could barely sleep, and the next four days found him scarcely able to crawl out of bed.

When he plucked up the courage to struggle to the chiropractor she found him leaning over to one side. Her examination and X-ray told her that Geoff was suffering from a jamming of the left facet joint between the third and fourth lumbar vertebrae. These are the small guiding joints that lie to the back of the vertebrae. She adjusted the facet joint, and Geoff left her feeling more upright. Three days later he was back at work. Seven years later Geoff has had no recurrence of back pain and his business is thriving.

LISA brought her two-week-old daughter to show her chiropractor, concerned that since her birth the baby's left foot had been turned more than 90 degrees outward compared with the right. He verified that there was no hip displacement and within a few minutes discovered an imbalance in the psoas muscles. Light pressure to a point at the side of the abdomen visibly brought the left foot back to its correct position within 30 seconds, and Lisa's daughter is now a lively six-year-old. She periodically takes her for a chiropractic check-up, strongly believing that her spine is every bit as important as her teeth.

JOAN always dreaded the onset of her monthly periods as they were not only very heavy but had given her agonizing pain ever since she was 14, and she often had to stay home from her work as a secretary. However, when she consulted her chiropractor it was not for these symptoms but for a stiff neck. She had woken two mornings before in agony, having turned awkwardly during her sleep. The chiropractor learned of her period problems while taking the case history, and resolved to thoroughly check her low back as well as her neck. A simple neck problem was solved with pressure to the neck muscles and with a special resisted exercise that was followed by one effective adjustment. However, a long-standing problem between her fifth lumbar vertebra and sacrum had led to a number of soft tissue changes in the area, and the chiropractor adjusted the fifth lumbar vertebra on several occasions. Joan's next two periods were pain-free, but she suffered pain again the following month. She has now found that a visit to her chiropractor every three months keeps her free of pain, bloating, and heavy periods, and she has not lost a day from work for nearly four years.

TED, 54, had suffered with back and leg pain for over a year and his employers had moved him from his job as a plumber to less demanding work in their stores. What particularly worried Ted was that for several weeks he had been tripping over his bad foot and was unable to lift it fully at the ankle. His doctor and a consultant at the hospital had told him it was arthritis and had sent him for physiotherapy. A friend at work had been trying to persuade him to visit a chiropractor for several months, but Ted was scared. His doctor had told him that chiropractors were untrained and dangerous, and Ted did not want to offend him. When traction to his lower back appeared to accelerate the foot-drop Ted became desperate. Feeling he had nothing to lose he plucked up courage and asked his friend for the chiropractor's telephone number.

The chiropractor tried to have the hospital X-rays sent to him but this was refused. Reluctantly he X-rayed Ted again, and found that the fifth vertebra had developed a spondylolisthesis.

It had slipped forward as a result of postural stress, causing wear and tear at the facet joints at the back of the vertebra. An adjustment was carefully chosen which would not strain the worn joints. Ted was placed on his back with his knees up whilst the chiropractor first rocked him gently and then delivered a light downward adjustment. Ted was surprised that there was no click, as his friend had told him to expect one. The chiropractor followed this with an adjustment to the neck, pressure on several postural muscles, advice on diet, posture, and giving up cigarettes, and a series of exercises.

There was no change for the first five visits, and on one occasion Ted had felt decidedly worse. He had followed the instructions to the letter, and his wife had started to chide him for going to 'an unqualified quack'. His friend at work had told him to persist as he knew that the chiropractor would say if he felt he could not help. On the next visit Ted voiced his concern, and although the chiropractor would not guarantee a favourable outcome he explained to Ted how the spine was now moving more naturally and asked Ted to allow him four more treatments. Two weeks later Ted's persistence had begun to pay dividends. The back pain was lifting, and the leg only ached if provoked by careless movement. Within another month strength had begun to return to the foot. Ted is now back at work as a plumber and is free of pain, although he controls his weight with a careful diet, continues his postural exercises, and avoids crouching down for long periods.

MERVIN was 34. He had a job in a night-club as a bouncer. One night he evicted one reveller for abusive behaviour. When he went home he was set upon from behind by six thugs who left him unconscious in an alley.

After two nights in hospital Mervin discharged himself and was back at work, apparently no worse for wear. About two months later he developed back pain and sciatica. His doctor gave him painkillers and told him it was from his past injuries. The pain got worse. Over the next six weeks he visited the doctor four times. Eventually an appointment was made to see an orthopaedic consultant two months later.

As Mervin was by now unable to sleep he went to a manipulator. After four manipulations he was in agony and decided to try a chiropractor. She X-rayed him and referred him to his medical doctor. Being on good terms with the local medical practice she phoned them and reported her findings. Seven weeks later Mervin died of cancer, but the prompt action taken by his chiropractor had made those last weeks more comfortable, as he responded well to the painkilling medication prescribed by his doctors.

EMILY was an independent woman of 92 and knew how to live life to the full. Having washed her curtains she was reaching up to rehang them when she felt her back give a loud crack, and pain came shortly afterwards. Her daughter took her to see her chiropractor, who examined and X-rayed her. The chiropractor diagnosed strain of a very unstable lumbar joint, and as the X-rays showed extensive osteoarthritis and bone thinning he chose a very rapid light adjustment that involved no twisting or straining of the back, massaged the muscles either side of the spine, and lay her on wedged blocks to gently level up the bones of her pelvis. Two weeks later Emily was mowing her lawn and cleaning her windows, having been painfree since that first visit.

ANN's morning chore was to drive the children to school before going on to her job as an accountant. Running behind schedule she didn't think when bending to raise the garage door. As she came up she forgot she was twisted and dropped to her knees in agony. Three days later her neighbour drove her to a chiropractor.

The chiropractor took the case history and examined Ann carefully. He noted that she had suffered constipation for about four years, following the birth of her last child. He chose not to X-ray Ann as her last monthly period was more than ten days previous and there was a chance she could be pregnant. Nevertheless he diagnosed an acute lower lumbar sprain related to a longstanding locking of the pelvis. He laid her on her right side and adjusted the left sacro-iliac joint, which gave a loud crunch. He also adjusted a locked second–third lumbar joint and her neck. Although she felt sore the next day her movements were freer, she was at last able to sit comfortably, and she experienced a good bowel movement. She suffered another bout of pain six months later, again after careless lifting, but this also responded to adjustment. An X-ray confirmed early wear and tear and instability between the fourth and fifth lumbar vertebrae. Ann now visits her chiropractor whenever she feels her back tightening up, and has remained clear of constipation for most of the time since that first chiropractic adjustment more than two years previously.

ALBERT had suffered chronic back pain for over fifteen years. He had tried everything and everybody, orthodox and unorthodox. The corset he wore to support his low back didn't really help, but he had worn one for the last thirteen years.

When a young chiropractor moved to his town someone suggested Albert go to see her. Even though he was by now quite cynical, Albert had never heard of a chiropractor and thought he would give her a try. She examined and X-rayed him, diagnosing lumbo-sacral instability related to an abnormally formed lower spine and a long-standing jamming of the right sacro-iliac joint. She adjusted him every other day for two weeks, whereupon Albert began to wake in the mornings with less pain and stiffness. Then she adjusted him twice a week for a month. Within four months Albert was discharged with an exercise programme and instructions to call if stiffness returned. He goes for a check-up every three months, has incinerated his corset, and has remained virtually painfree ever since.

FREDA had experienced considerable back pain when carrying her first child, and had suffered a long and arduous labour. Although her pain had left her several months after the birth, she dreaded the thought of another pregnancy. Two years later she conceived again. When her back pain returned she followed the advice of her best friend and went to her local chiropractor. He carefully examined her but took no X-rays. He noted several lumbar joints were restricted in certain movements and others were becoming too mobile. This joint mobility was being aided by Freda's production of the hormone relaxin, which allows the pelvic ligaments to stretch ready for the birth process. In addition, Freda's new posture was causing her to lean backwards, placing strain on the facet (guiding) joints which lie at the back of the spine. The chiropractor adjusted the restricted vertebrae and continued to monitor Freda's progress every two weeks. She was amazed to remain so free of back pain during the rest of her pregnancy and subsequent labour, and returned to her chiropractor after the birth not only for a check on her own spine but so he could screen her two young children. She has since had her third child, and enjoyed a comfortable pregnancy throughout.

MIDDLE AND UPPER BACK PROBLEMS

GEORGE was terrified he had heart problems. His father had suffered angina for twenty years and he knew he was overweight. At times his chest pains kept him awake at night, and certain movements anguished him during the day. His life as an insurance agent was stressful, and he thought his days were numbered. His doctor noted George's moderately high blood-pressure, gave him antihypertensive tablets, but told him his heart sounded normal. Because he still suffered pain George didn't fully believe him.

George's job involved a lot of driving and getting in and out of the car. He started to develop neck and shoulder pain, and one of his clients told him to see a chiropractor. George described his life-style and all his symptoms, confiding his fears about a heart attack. The chiropractor checked his eyes with an ophthalmo-scope, listened to his heart, and took his blood pressure and pulse. There were minor signs of hardened arteries, but George's heart sounded as strong as an ox and his blood pressure was not dangerously high. He noted a small problem in the upper neck, but suspected a restriction of the upper thoracic vertebrae could be responsible not only for the neck and shoulder pain but also for the chest pains. The first thoracic vertebra appeared to have rotated to one side. X-rays showed a normal heart shape and size and a normal lung field. There were degenerative changes to the mid-thoracic vertebrae, and a reversal of the normal thoracic curve higher up, but that apparent deviation of the first vertebra was not a displacement at all but a harmless irregularity of one of its bony projections, present since birth. There was no need to adjust that, and if it had been manipulated it could have triggered an unnecessary attack of pain. Instead, the chiropractor turned George onto his back, cupped his hand over the fifth thoracic vertebra, and crossed George's arms over his chest. As George breathed out and brought his chin down to his chest he felt the chiropractor drop lightly onto him with a pop. As he sat up he could already feel greater neck movement. This was improved further with a neck adjustment. George was told to go home, take the next day, a Friday, off work, and to enjoy a relaxed weekend. By Monday his chest pains had gone, a week later the neck and shoulders were clear, and a month later the blood pressure reading was well into normal range. The chiropractor sent him back to his doctor to re-evaluate medication. He was taken off drugs and his blood pressure remains sound. George has followed a diet given by his chiropractor, has lost weight, and has taken up controlled exercise which he enjoys.

BEVERLEY was 14 when her mother brought her to a chiropractor with scoliosis. Beverley was quiet and shy, and hadn't socialized much at school since being told that she had a curved spine. The other children made fun of her and called her the hunchback of Notre Dame. The school doctor had sent her to a consultant. He warned he might have to prescribe a brace if things got any worse, and Beverley was convinced she was a freak. She threw herself into her studies to forget her problems.

Her chiropractor listened carefully to the story and examined Beverley. She explained to her that a scoliosis was fairly common in children of her age, and in no way should Beverley feel abnormal or a freak. She gave her several exercises to do regularly, advised on diet and relaxation, suggested a modern Scandinavian Balans style chair and desk for homework, and adjusted several joints of her spine. She gave no promises to Beverley's mother, explained that many scolioses resolve on their own, and emphasized that stress and worry often make things worse, whilst love and home security help boost a child. She agreed to check Beverley's back regularly, and adjusted her a number of times over the coming months. As Beverley began to relax her confidence returned and her spine stabilized. She is now a very confident dental nurse of 20.

RICHARD was enjoying his third year at university and was actively involved in rowing. Two weeks before an important boat race he developed excruciating rib pain, could not take a deep breath, and was forced to stop training. The coach suggested he visit a chiropractor.

Richard's problem was visible the moment he removed his shirt. Having spent so much time as a left-sided oarsman he had overdeveloped his muscles on the left whilst neglecting those on the right. He had further compensated by developing a general curve and twist in his spine. The rowing action was affecting the normal mechanics of Richard's spine, so that whenever he took up the strain of the oar he leant away, twisted the upper spine backwards on the right, and overloaded himself. The immediate problem was resolved within a couple of days and Richard was given exercises to develop the weaker side and instructions on improving his rowing technique. Although his boat failed to qualify for the finals, Richard carried on rowing and his rib pain has never returned.

NECK PROBLEMS

JANET, who was 32, had suffered from headaches ever since she was 17. Her doctor believed it to be a hormonal problem and at first told her it would go away when she started a family. At 24 Janet became a mother, but apart from a slight reduction in frequency and severity during her pregnancy there was no genuine change. In the five years that followed Janet tried a number of alternative therapies, but with no lasting results. At one time she thought that careful dietary control was helping her by eliminating certain foods, but she still suffered a couple of bad headaches most months, and had recently been experiencing ringing in her ears and a general muzziness.

When she visited a chiropractor he took her through her case history in great detail and emphasized accidents and injuries, but Janet could remember no incidents at all. He examined her neck and with his fingers detected a sensitive fullness at the base of her skull, which coincided with a restriction of its normal rocking movement on the right. The first vertebra appeared more prominent there, and this was confirmed by X-ray. The chiropractor completed his examination with tests for the cranial nerves, and he checked the eyes with an ophthalmoscope, read the blood pressure, and performed other manual tests before telling Janet he had found a possible cause for her headaches in the faulty atlas vertebra. Janet was a little reluctant, as she had received neck manipulation unsuccessfully in the past, but she agreed to a series of six treatments.

The chiropractor placed Janet on her left side with a specially designed mechanical pillow under her head. He set a spring on this and carefully placed the edge of his wrist over her top vertebra. This was reinforced by the left hand, and in a split second the toggle recoil adjustment was over. The pre-set spring gave way as the pillow dropped about half an inch, and Janet was experiencing a warm glow over her head and hands. He could have delivered the toggle adjustment without the special pillow, but he found it helped him measure more accurately the direction, torque, and strength of his adjustment.

When Janet returned for her second appointment she reported that her hearing was more acute, she had lost the ringing noise, – or tinnitus – in her ears, and her breathing was freer. She had suffered sinus congestion for as long as she could remember and had learned to live with it, but for the two days following treatment she felt exhausted and her nasal passages were flooded with fluid. When this ceased she felt completely invigorated, and returned for her second treatment looking radiant. With the exception of mild muzzy headaches related to late nights or stress Janet has been clear of her old head pain now for over four years; she has also been clear of tinnitus, and her nasal passages have not troubled her.

BERNARD had enjoyed playing bowls for more than twenty years, and since retiring from his bicycle shop a year ago had lived for the sport. Shortly after retiring he began to experience arm pain and weakness, and now could barely hold the wood. He started to drop things at home, could no longer open a jar or tin, and constantly had to shake his right hand to rid himself of numbing pins and needles. Restful sleep was a thing of the past as Bernard kept having to shake his arm and hang it out of the bed every 15 or 20 minutes. His doctor tried to manipulate the neck, but this had only made Bernard dizzy and nauseous and increased the pain. Bernard was sent away with tablets for arthritis and was told to learn to live with it.

The chiropractor found Bernard despondent. He had only gone to the clinic to prove a friend wrong. She had badgered him at the bowls club until he complied just to keep her quiet. His doctor had told him not to have chiropractic treatment as it was dangerous. Having already experienced manipulation Bernard at first wanted an opinion only but no treatment.

The chiropractor could tell that Bernard suffered from advanced cervical spondylosis (neck arthritis) and that there was considerable neck restriction. Even quite small movements induced a shooting arm pain. Some neck movements made Bernard dizzy. The X-rays confirmed that arthritic changes to the neck had reached an advanced stage. They also showed the presence of a rare abnormal joint between the tip of the atlas and the skull itself, present since birth. Only very careful neck adjustment would be possible, and taking full account of the unusual mechanics that this joint created the chiropractor devised an approach that was risk-free and founded on his specialist knowledge. Bernard has now been free of pain night and day for more than six months and continues to enjoy bowls.

SAMMY was small for his age and had been picked on at school. He had therefore taken up one of the martial arts and by the age of twelve had become proficient and could look after himself well. Whilst waiting for the school bus he was attacked from behind by four 16-year-olds and caught unawares. The next morning his mother brought him to her chiropractor with a wry neck. Severe pain restricted all movement in every direction. After a thorough case history, examination, and elimination of other possibilities Sammy was diagnosed as suffering from acute torticollis from his injuries, and with difficulty was coaxed onto his back. For the next five minutes he tensed, held and relaxed his muscles in turn whilst the chiropractor's firm hands prevented even the slightest movement. After these exercises Sammy found he could move his head considerably more to the left, and the chiropractor decided it was safe to try a short sharp adjustment in that direction.

When Sammy left shortly afterwards about 50 per cent of his neck movement had been restored. This was maintained over the next 24 hours, and a follow-up treatment the following day brought even more mobility. Sammy's neck movements were full and pain-free within four days, in spite of his proud assertion that he had given his assailants a lesson they would never forget.

TOM was a self-employed bricklayer aged 37, and depended on working hard during the summer months to make up for the slack winter period. Towards the end of May he was having difficulty gripping his trowel, and the action of striking bricks and blocks to shape them gave a sharp electric-shock-like pain that made him drop the trowel. By the end of June he was behind with work and had to subcontract to another bricklayer, even though he would now make a loss on the job. Pain, numbness, or pins and needles were with him day and night, and his doctor prescribed rest and muscle relaxants and arranged for him to see an orthopaedic surgeon in September. It was expected that by December the surgeon would operate to decompress the carpal tunnel in Tom's right wrist.

When Tom visited the chiropractor at the end of July he was desperately worried about paying his bills as he had no sickness insurance to cover him. The chiropractor not only confirmed the carpal tunnel diagnosis with several tests, but also found a locking of vertebrae both at the top and bottom of the neck. She adjusted these areas, and also a problem in the lumbar spine. She also explained how irritation from the neck could alter the pain threshold of nerves leading to the arm, and showed an area of spondylosis (arthritis) on the X-ray which was contributing to the situation. Within two treatments Tom was experiencing some symptomless periods, but he could still not grip without pain. Progress continued over the next four weeks and by the end of August he was back at work. He experienced a couple of short relapses during the next two busy months but paid his bills and kept his business going. Six years later he still visits his chiropractor if he feels the slightest hint of pain, but he has not lost a day's work since then.

JANE's frozen shoulder had troubled her for several months and her medical doctor had told her she would have to live with it until it cleared on its own. She was particularly frustrated, for during the 62 years of her life she had never really experienced any illness, and this unaccustomed pain and restriction was getting her down. The great love of her life was golf, but her shoulder restriction gave her agony when she forced herself to play. She couldn't even comb her hair or do up her bra strap, and she had to rely on assistance from her husband. It was he who persuaded her to visit the local chiropractor.

He examined Jane and after taking an X-ray showed her on the film the spot where arthritis in the neck was irritating a nerve that governed the shoulder muscles. He explained that often shoulder restriction remained for some months in cases of shoulder Retractile Capsulitis, but that chiropractic adjustment was usually successful in removing the pain associated with it. After one adjustment Jane noticed a change in the symptoms. A week later she could comb her hair without pain, and soon could dress herself unaided. Exercises were gradually helping to clear adhesions in the joint and, although there was pain if she suddenly forgot herself and stretched the shoulder to extremes, it was much more tolerable and she began to feel like her old self.

It was a further three months before she was in top form on the golfing green, but she is sure that it was her chiropractic treatment that got her there more quickly and painlessly than the tablets her medical doctor had prescribed.

SARAH's neck pain had troubled her on and off for three years and had affected her ability to play the church organ on Sundays. She enjoyed the keyboard and usually practised two or three hours each day, especially since her children had left home. However, at the end of each session her shoulders had tightened, a headache threatened, and her neck hurt her. A friend in her church congregation referred her to a local chiropractor, who gave her a thorough examination. He discovered an area in her neck that was restricted and another in her thoracic spine. X-rays demonstrated the wear and tear this had caused and also two vertebrae that had been fused from birth. Armed with this information her chiropractor was able to devise the best pain-free adjustment, and accompanied this with a series of soft tissue mobilizations and exercises. Within a month Sarah was free of pain, and although she visits her chiropractor for an occasional treatment she rarely suffers any symptoms and they are always short-lived.

TONY had suffered the misfortune of being a passenger in two traffic accidents in four months. The first had been fairly minor, and left him with a sore neck for about a week. The second was a head-on collision that was more serious, giving him a classic whiplash injury. Tony was still at school, but in two months' time he was due to take the examinations needed for a place at university. Hospital X-rays taken at the time had revealed injury, and doctors had sent him home with a soft neck-collar.

The initial symptoms settled down within four days, but four weeks later they returned with a vengeance. Not only was there severe pain when Tony bent his head to study or write notes, but his headaches were intolerable. Once or twice his vision had become disturbed, and he entered into a deep depression. His first examinations were only three weeks away, yet he could not concentrate for more than a few moments at a time. He knew he would fail in spite of all his hard work and the confidence his teachers had placed in him.

When his father brought Tony to the chiropractor there was only a week to go and Tony had given up hope. After examining neck movement the chiropractor noted a very unstable joint and so X-rayed him, first looking straight ahead, then with the head held forwards, and finally with the neck stretched backwards. The X-ray showed nothing of note with the head in a neutral position, but when the head was bent forwards a massive displacement of one vertebra was clearly visible.

A series of treatments was given which concentrated on loosening the upper thoracic spine as well as delivering a specific neck adjustment. Tony was shown how to apply ice-packs at home, and was told to wear the soft collar at night during this critical time. Although not out of pain he entered his first examination feeling more confident, and as he progressed through these he found himself more able to cope. His grades were not as good as he or his teachers had hoped, but they were sufficient to guarantee Tony a place at university.

CHRISTINA had been suffering exhaustion for several months and she had sought help from her family medical physician. He ascribed the symptoms to the effects of stress, as Christina had been going through problems with her two teenage daughters for over a year, and the family was experiencing financial problems. He therefore prescribed anti-depressants.

Lethargy continued to lower Christina's spirit and she began to put on weight in spite of eating very little. Her hair started to become lifeless, brittle, and coarse, and her face was puffy. Her skin began to scale in places and was very dry. As she became more obese she developed low-back pain, and a friend persuaded her to visit a chiropractor.

The chiropractor took a detailed case history and appeared more interested in Christina's lethargic symptoms than her low-back problem. She took a sample of Christina's blood and sent it for analysis. Meanwhile she examined her spine thoroughly and reported finding restriction not only in movements of the low back but at two places in the neck. The atlas vertebra at the top of the neck was adjusted, with Christina sitting back comfortably in a specially designed tilting chiropractic chair. The chiropractor decided not to adjust any other vertebra on this occasion, and reported an improvement in movement throughout the spine afterwards.

When Christina returned for her second treatment she was feeling much better in herself and her low back was easier. The chiropractor now had the results of Christina's blood test which pointed to a sluggish thyroid gland, and she explained that some cases of thyroid malfunction can be attributed to subluxations in the spine. Christina was given the option of asking her medical doctor for a course of thyroid hormones, but the chiropractor offered to monitor her symptoms while she corrected faulty spinal movement. If the symptoms worsened or persisted for a month then she would refer Christina for medical care.

Christina's low-back pain had cleared within a week, and within a month her puffiness and dry skin had gone. Her full level of energy returned, and her hair started to shine again. Before discharging her two months later the chiropractor took another blood test, and this showed her thyroid hormone levels to be quite normal again. Christina is sure that if she had not had chiropractic treatment she would have had to take thyroxine tablets for a very long time.

Chapter 4

PREVENTION IS BETTER THAN CURE

The Doctor of the future will give no medicine, but will interest his patients in the care of the human frame in diet and in the cause and prevention of disease. *Thomas A. Edison* (1847–1931)

The great advances made this century in health care have been founded upon concepts of preventative public health developed during the nineteeth century. Two centuries ago life expectancy was 32 years, and 10 per cent of children died within their first year. Clean water supplies and efficient sewage disposal have slashed child mortality to one death in 500, and have extended life expectancy way beyond the biblical three score years and ten. There have been great advances in drug therapy and surgery with the advent of antibiotics and dramatic organ transplants. These have tended to steal the limelight in the last fifty years, detracting from the immense strides made by preventative medicine in the last one hundred and fifty years. It is the advances in preventative care which have quietly laid the true foundation for the twentieth century's claim to be the healthiest in the history of the Western world. Preventative medicine has been dwarfed to such an extent by the media dramas of medicine's 'battle' against the 'armies' of disease that modern illnesses have crept upon as unawares, closely allied to a poor appreciation of the dangers of inadequate diet, stress, and environmental pollution. As we approach the next millenium let us hope we are capable of building health upon concepts of personal preventative care.

Notions of prevention are not new to this or to previous ages. They are clearly laid down in the Talmud and Bible, and are to be found in ancient Arabic, Indian, and Chinese writings. Hippocrates placed great store on prevention, laying down criteria for town planning in his treatise *Airs, Waters, Places*, and for personal hygiene, diet, exercise, and mental health in many of his other works. These axioms remain unchallenged more than two thousand years later.

DIET

The body is unlike any other machine in that it has the innate capacity to regenerate itself. Cells wear out and die in their millions every day, yet they are carried away, broken down, reprocessed, and replaced. Waste matter is ejected from the bowels, bladder, lungs, and skin and new materials are taken in as food, to be broken down into tiny substances that will provide energy, chemical catalysts, and new building blocks for the growth or regeneration processes. If we ingest foods that have much of their goodness cooked or processed out of them then regeneration is impaired and our bodies suffer. If we swamp our food with useless or harmful colourings or preservatives then we risk interfering with nature's delicate biochemical processes.

Even natural foods possess some toxic elements, but mankind's evolutionary journey has equipped organs such as the liver to detoxify them effectively. These same pathways enable us to deal with most modern food additives, so that convenience or 'junk' foods eaten in moderation usually do us little harm. However, those who rely on processed foods or who do not vary their diet impair their body's regenerative ability and leave themselves open to colds, infections, tiredness, irritability, and a myriad of conditions associated with ill health. The saying, 'You are what you eat' is one to be heeded. A diet low in refined flour and sugars, high in natural fibre from raw or lightly cooked vegetables and fruit, and balanced with a wide variety of proteins obtainable from eggs, fish, meat, or pulses is one to be striven after, and one we ignore at our own and our family's peril.

Water intake is frequently overlooked. The body requires six to eight large glasses a day to help flush the kidneys and bowels and compensate for fluids lost from the lungs and skin. Water helps purify the system and assists the passage of waste through the intestines, and many cases of constipation are helped by attention to water intake. Headaches and other signs of toxicity may be eliminated by effectively flushing the kidneys. Even fluid retention can be reduced by increasing fluid intake for, although this may appear paradoxical, the intake of pure water flushes out through the kidneys the body salts that are responsible for over-retention; this is the reason why table salt should not be added to food.

Do not rely on cups of tea or coffee to provide your fluid intake. Apart from introducing toxic substances, they fail to act as effectively in flushing the system as pure water. It is wise to initiate the cleansing process every day with a glass of water at room temperature at least 15 minutes before you have breakfast. To aid digestion after a meal sipping a cup of hot water can be a most pleasant way of raising your fluid intake.

EXERCISE

Those who try to start their car after a long holiday, or their motor-lawnmower in the first warm days of spring, will have experienced the coughing and spluttering of an engine struggling to get back to life after a period of inactivity. If we neglect to exercise our bodies our lungs fail to fully expand, our arteries clog up with cholesterol, our muscles become flaccid, our body tissues and organs function below par, we put on weight, and we generally fall out of condition. Not only does exercise get our body working again, but it cleanses us internally, brings the fuel of oxygen to every cell of the body, improves our biochemical and regenerative processes, revitalizes us in body and mind, and makes us feel really good.

Exercise should be chosen for enjoyment and not be treated as drudgery. Some enjoy competitive sports. Others like to set themselves personal targets to reach, maintain, and improve; these can be in running, walking, swimming, horse-riding, cycling, gymnastics or yoga, amongst many others – there is much to choose from. Existing back problems may limit you and your chiropractor may advise you to avoid sports such as squash, where you risk twisting and overreaching your spine. Swimming, which is generally an excellent all-round toning exercise, may trigger off a bout of neck pain if you have a problem there. When running you should avoid hard jarring surfaces, and should make sure that your footwear is sufficient to absorb the stress as your feet strike the ground.

To be really effective an exercise programme should be

followed no less than three times a week for 30 minutes each session. The first five minutes is a warm-up to stretch and prepare muscles and to gradually raise the heart rate. Twenty minutes of sustained exercise should follow, during which the heart should beat at a rate of about 120 to 130 pulses per minute for a good five minutes. Continuous exercise during this time keeps oxygen pumping through the system, until the final five minute phase when reduced activity introduces the cooling down process. It must be reiterated that you should never go 'cold' into vigorous exercise, for it will lay you wide open to muscle, ligament, or joint injuries and strains. If you have any history of heart disease or have become severely out of condition you must first have a cardiovascular check-up before introducing yourself very gradually to such an exercise programme. Never try to make up for lost time by premature exertion. Time taken in slowly building up stamina and natural resistance is time well spent.

FRESH AIR

Exercise helps to bring oxygen to help regenerate the body, but other forces can hinder this process. Smoking, whether directly through your own habit, or indirectly through sharing a smoke-filled office or living room, will inhibit oxygen transfer. So do car exhaust fumes and other environmental pollutants. If you live in a heavily-polluted city environment you can try to remedy the situation with air filtration and an ionizer, but you should also use every opportunity to enjoy fresh country air. If you smoke you should recognize it as a killer, not necessarily because it is a major cause of cancer, but primarily because it is more likely to induce heart disease than any other factor.

RELAXATION

Sleep is nature's way of closing down the physical and mental consciousness so that repair and reconditioning can occur without hindrance. Individuals vary in their needs, but your body will tell you by experience the number of hours of sleep required to enable you to awake alert and refreshed. There are many factors which intervene to influence the quality of sleep. Stress patterns may interfere with the process, so that whether you have two or ten hours of sleep these may be marred by deep underlying troubles which rob you of power and vitality during waking hours. Indeed it is the quality and not the quantity of sleep which is important, and it is possible for most of us to train ourselves down from eight to six or less hours each night provided these are filled with the right type of sleep.

Recognition of the causes of stress is important in that it takes away fear of the unknown. This does not mean that we must all psychoanalyse ourselves to get to the bottom of our tensions; most of us will uncover the causes if we allow ourselves time for quiet contemplation. In some cases we can eliminate the causes of stress directly, but frequently we find ourselves in situations we can do little to alter, other than by recognizing and accepting the source, and by mitigating the effects of anxiety through simple mental relaxation techniques. Such exercises are so easy that they can be adopted by anyone prepared to give themselves a little time and a little patience.

The principle of most relaxation techniques relies on reversing the tension process. Anxiety activates the postural muscles in a primitive 'fight or flight' response. Relaxation starts by consciously letting go of these muscle tensions. As the body relaxes, its pre-set biological programming reciprocates by relaxing the mind. By learning to relax your body and then calming your mind you can reach a state of mental tranquillity which will persist into your physical activites.

There are a number of good books and tapes available on the subject of managing stress through relaxation techniques, and these can be most helpful. A comfortable but not sleep-inducing position is chosen and a conscious effort is made to go through an inventory, contracting and then relaxing areas of the body in turn until physical calm has been reached. Facial muscles reflect the emotional state, and when you have relaxed these you are ready to translate that state of physical calm into one of mental calm. Usually this is done in rhythm with breathing, so that as you breath out you let yourself go, allowing yourself with every breath to go deeper and deeper, as you ease further and further into a state of quiet harmony. Here you may transfer your mind to a place of natural peace and tranquillity, perhaps a burbling brook, a deserted sea shore, a quiet meadow, or a hill-top. At this stage healing of the mind and the emotions begins. Everyone can reach that healthful state, given time, and once relaxation has been experienced you will look forward to the next 15 or 20 minute session you have set aside once or twice in your daily routine. In the early stages patience and persistence may be required before you reach your goal, and you should not be disappointed if it takes a little time. Everyone can achieve it, and whether you believe you suffer stress or not, with the right help you can learn mental relaxation techniques which will enrich the quality of your life, promoting health and longevity.

If self-help brings only a limited response, then professional counselling with a qualified therapist will often overcome the innate barrier that blocks many people. Others find that various forms of meditation or prayer bring them an inner peace, but whichever road you choose to take to banish stress it will require an active decision on your part to set aside time during the day for the purpose. Once the will is there, you will find the way.

POSTURE

Back and neck strain can often be attributed to weakening of the muscles and ligaments brought on by poor posture. When the body is properly balanced the muscle tone on one side of a joint or series of joints is counterbalanced by the tone on the opposite side. If this does not occur, the muscles on one side become overloaded and fatigue rapidly, causing harmful lengthening of the ligaments. Once a ligament has been lengthened it can no longer effectively fulfil its function, and fails to prevent its own joint from overreaching. Joint strain and muscle tearing then occur.

As a ready guide to your posture, stand facing a wall, just touching it with your toes. If your abdomen touches the wall you are at great risk from overloading the lumbar spine and slouching the shoulders. Only your chest should touch the wall, and nothing else, except perhaps the tip of your nose. Turn around. Stand with your heels, calf muscles, buttocks, shoulder-blades, and head in contact with the wall. Tense your buttock muscles so as to tilt the pelvis and flatten the hollow of your back. If you can pass the flat of your hand between the hollow and the wall, correction of your sway-back posture is required. Finally, turn and face a full-length mirror. Your shoulders and hips should be level. If either side is higher, an imbalance exists.

Once a weakness has been identified, try to determine the cause. Poor posture may be due to weak muscle tone, lack of exercise, overweight, occupational habits or strains, incorrect sleeping or sitting positions, depression, injury, or birth or growing defects. Think carefully of the possible causes so that you can give your chiropractor clues that may help to reverse this damaging process. Often only you can provide those clues, for no one else follows your movements 24 hours a day, every day.

CORRECT SITTING

Make sure that you sit well back in a chair with your buttocks and lumbar spine firmly supported by the chair back, and your thighs supported by the length of the seat. You may cross your legs at the ankle, but never at the knees – as you cross one thigh over the other you create a pelvic imbalance that can jam the sacro-iliac joints or overload the lumbar spine. Do not let the low back slump, as this pushes the buttocks and shoulders forward, stretching ligaments and joints and in time damaging your posture. If you feel tired do not allow yourself to slide into sleep on the floor or in a chair or sofa but take yourself off to bed. Sleeping in chairs overstretches the low back, pushes the head forward, and risks neck strain. Choose chairs that support your back and avoid soft reclining chairs that offer no back support or require a real effort to get out of. If it is too late to change your chairs, purchase a movable back support or roll up a bath towel to support your lumbar spine. The last two decades have seen the evolution of ergonomically designed Balans furniture from Scandinavia. The seat itself is set at a slight angle and the thighs and buttocks are so balanced that the perfect sitting posture is adopted with no effort. Gravity alone provides lumbar support, so that the chair has no back at all yet remains restful and comforting. There are a number of seat wedges commercially available which will convert a conventional chair seat to the optimum sitting angle.

When driving, ensure that your lumbar spine and thighs are well supported, that your feet are not too far from the pedal controls, that your head is comfortably balanced, and that your arms are close enough to the steering wheel but not cramped. You will find that as you press your back firmly against the lumbar support your head and shoulders straighten. If your

Sitting

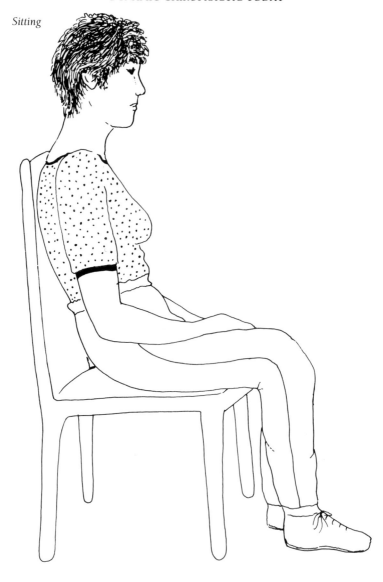

Sitting in the slumped position forces open the lumbar facet joints and pressurizes the discs. The shoulders and head ride forwards and the body tires rapidly

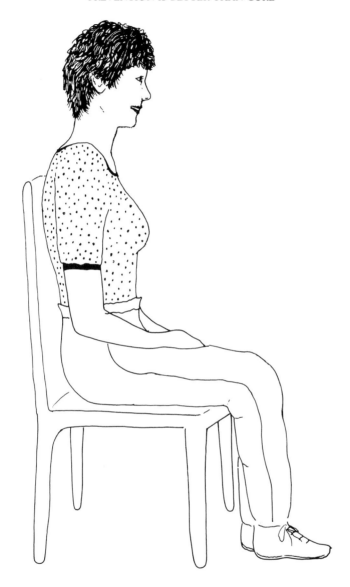

Sitting with the buttocks pressed against the back of the chair allows the trunk, shoulders and head to adopt a more balanced position, reducing strain on the neck and aiding concentration. The thigh muscles are not in balance in a conventional chair and the buttocks tend to ride forwards to compensate unless a conscious effort is made to maintain the position

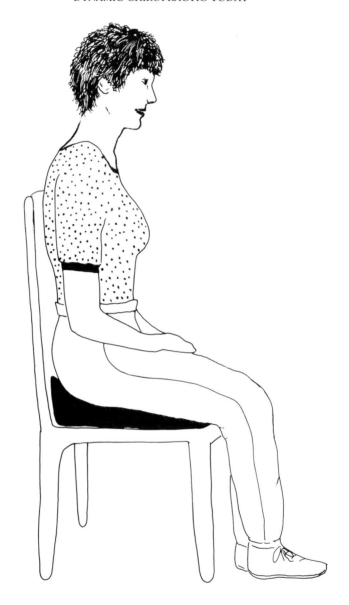

A portable seat wedge is a cheap and effective means of converting an upright chair into one which is comfortable for long periods of time. It allows the correct spinal position to be matched by a balanced thigh and pelvic posture. Scandinavian Balans furniture adopts this principle into its designs

buttocks slide forward, your shoulders slump, your head rides forward, and your chin tilts upward. You will rapidly tire in this position, and alertness will be lost. If your car seat lacks a lumbar support, make your own with a small cushion or a tightly wrapped towel or, better still, purchase a support to suit your build. This can then be taken from seat to seat whether you are driving or just travelling as a passenger.

If you are too tall to sit correctly you should change your seat or your car, especially if you drive long distances for a living. Even smooth motorway driving picks up minute road vibrations which, in the slumped position, imperceptibly tug at over-stretched ligaments. When you reach your destination those first staggering steps are telling you to support your lumbar spine.

If, in spite of lumbar support, long journeys still give you back pain, discipline yourself to stop every 30 minutes. Get out of the car and stretch your legs for about 5 minutes before driving on. The temptation to carry on driving another 5 minutes is always there, especially if there is a lot of freight on the roads, but strict self-discipline pays handsome dividends; it not only saves you pain but keeps you on the road and working.

On arriving at your destination take care how you get out of the car – whether you are driving or a passenger. Open the door, and keeping your knees together use your arms and not your back to ease yourself around on your buttocks until you can place both feet on the ground. Then stand up smoothly and evenly without bending or twisting to either side.

RECLINING AND SLEEPING

When reclining or sleeping choose a firm surface that supports you without sagging yet yields at pressure points to allow even support. As a rough guide this can be represented as 4 inches (10 cm) of dense foam rubber, but individuals vary in their needs according to their weight and stature. A pillow should also be provided to support the neck. Again variations exist between individuals, but it is rare that more than one pillow is required. The pillow should be tucked well into the neck so that cervical spinal alignment is preserved in relation to the rest of the back. A special pillow with an in-built neck support helps maintain alignment throughout the night, but you can emulate this with a rolled up towel placed under the neck (although it can dislodge

Driving

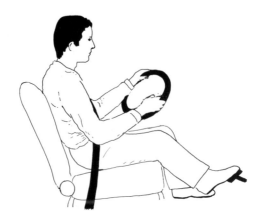

Inadequate lumbar support when driving leads to slumping, pushing the shoulders forward whilst extending the neck to look ahead. This rapidly leads to aching low back, shoulders, neck, head and arms, as well as to driver fatigue

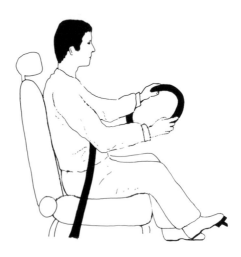

A seat with an adequate lumbar support maintains balanced thoracic and neck curves, reducing fatigue and aiding concentration. By supporting the lumbar region it reduces low-back pain. Ensure the seat is high enough at the back, especially if you are tall, and that you have a head restraint. Sit well back into the seat and support the length of the thighs

itself as you move during the night). If you use too many pillows, your head is pushed away from the mattress and therefore away from the spinal mid-line. Conversely, no pillow at all will also create distortion, especially if you spend most of the night on your side.

The most natural sleeping position is lying on your side with your knees together and drawn up slightly. The spine should not be rotated, so ensure you are side-lying and not twisting onto back or front with your torso. Ensure you have adequate neck support in this position so that your cervical vertebrae remain in line with the rest of the spine.

Lying on your back may also be satisfactory. However, a common postural weakness can allow the pelvis to rock forward in this position, increasing the lumbar curve and stressing the spine. If this is the case you will awake in pain and may have to draw up your knees, hugging them to your chest for five minutes before you can get out of bed painlessly. You will need to train yourself to sleep on your side until your posture has been corrected.

Certain positions create risks of their own. Lying in a hot bath with the head pushed forwards can not only create neck strain, but the heat can excessively loosen ligaments in the lumbar spine. Too much time spent relaxing in a hot bath after gardening or after long periods of stretching can create the problems you are trying to avoid, even though both the bath and the warmth are in themselves comforting. In these circumstances it is better to sit well back in a chair with a warm (not hot) hot water bottle firmly tucked into the small of the back to maintain the lumbar curve, and to avoid all lifting or twisting for the rest of the day.

Lying in bed with the head pushed forward reading or watching television can bring on neck strain, arthritic change, and eventually permanent damage, especially if it becomes a regular habit. Likewise, regularly lying on your abdomen not only reduces breathing capacity and cramps vital organs, but it accentuates lumbar and neck distortion patterns. For babies, lying face down in the prone position serves to develop the secondary neck and low-back curves and muscles required for the upright posture, and is an essential part of development. But in adults the curves are already there and the prone position exaggerates these, seriously weakening the spine. Many is the holidaymaker whose holiday has been ruined by back pain brought on by lying face down in the warm sun reading a book.

Lying on your side

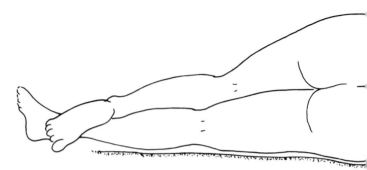

A mattress should support the pelvis whilst allowing some give in the pelvic and shoulder regions to maintain the neutral line of the spine. The pillow should support the neck so that the neutral line is preserved

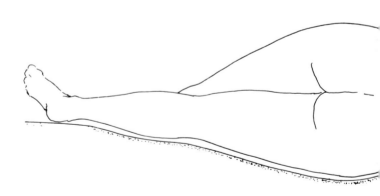

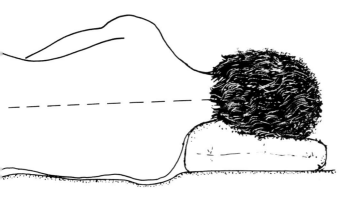

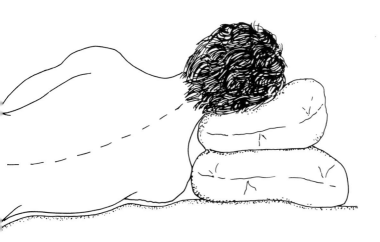

A mattress which is too soft tends to sag in the region of the pelvis, curving the lumbar spine. Too many pillows curve the upper thoracic and cervical spinal area

Lying on your back

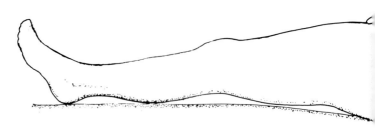

A firm mattress which supports the back should allow enough give for the buttocks and shoulders. Only one pillow should be used, primarily to support the neck rather than the head

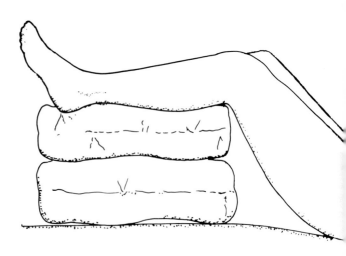

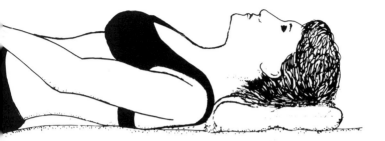

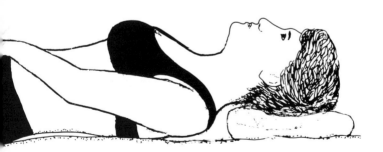

As the psoas muscle is stretched when lying on the back the natural lumbar curve is accentuated. This may cause pain. Lying with pillows supporting the knees flattens the curve and eases the pain

71

Most of us turn several times during the night from one position to another. Normally we do so painlessly. At times we may awake with searing neck pain, perhaps because we have used the head as a pivot whilst the shoulders turn us around. When turning in bed always try to lift the head from the pillow; even though you may not have full control during sleep, subconscious awareness of how strains occur often aids re-education.

When you awake in the morning try to avoid leaping out of bed. Instead, turn onto your side near the edge of the bed, draw up the knees so that your lower legs hang over the side, and gently push yourself up into the sitting position allowing the force of gravity on your legs to assist as a counterbalance. If you are in pain take your time before getting up from the sitting position. If you are in a lot of pain you may have to roll out of bed onto your knees, pushing yourself slowly upright from the kneeling position. Morning pain often indicates joint damage, inflammation, or degenerative changes. Pain that occurs during the day is often related to postural or occupational strains of muscles and ligaments.

SEX AND YOUR SPINE

A number of patients worry that love-making will upset their existing back problems but, with few exceptions, gentle love-making will reduce tensions, reinforce bonds with your partner, and relax the lumbar spine. If back pain does occur try to find a position which avoids provoking the spine, using a pillow to bolster the buttocks, thighs or spine if necessary. Often pain is brought on by stretching the spine too far backwards or by sudden exerted movement. Although excessive preparation can destroy spontaneity, an awareness by you and your partner of those positions or movements which provoke pain will help you avoid them, and so enable you to relax.

For those who do not suffer a bad back, love-making with a caring partner can not only bring emotional and stress-relieving rewards but can exercise the spine most beneficially. However, neck problems may occur if the head is extended too far back at times of heightened passion, and when you lie on your back avoid bending your head and neck backwards to take any weight.

BENDING AND LIFTING

When you are standing upright gravity ensures that your body weight is carried with the minimum of strain on your lumbar spine. When you bend forward the centre of gravity changes and the hips and pelvis act as the fulcrum of movement. The laws of physics teach us that the leverage created by the bending movement increases the load on the lower lumbar discs, so that pressure on these discs is around six times greater than when you are upright. If you then pick up a weight of ten pounds your lumbar discs must not only cope with your increased relative body weight but with an additional sixty pounds, until you reach the upright position again. If the lifted weight is held away from the body the load can be even greater, so weights should always be held as close to your body as possible.

When you lift an object, face it and place your feet either side of it. Keep the back straight and bend the hips and knees, lowering your body and arms to grasp it firmly. This ensures that the centre of gravity remains over the object to be lifted, minimizing the strain from the leverage effect. To help raise the weight with less effort use kinetic energy by co-ordinating a body drop, leg spring, and leg straightening in that order. It is important that you anticipate the weight, avoid excessively heavy objects, grip firmly, and raise the load smoothly and evenly without losing balance.

Studies have identified a 'creep effect' which causes the discs to compress measurably after a mere 15 seconds. Leaning forward, even with just your body weight, creates enough pressure to compromise your lumbar discs even in such a short space of time. If you must lean forward for longer, make sure that you rest your chest or abdomen on a supporting surface so that strain is taken away from the lumber spine.

Strong abdominal muscles are essential if you bend or lift. Their contraction raises pressure within the thorax and abdomen, thereby cushioning the strain. Loads on the spine can be reduced by 25 per cent with healthy abdominal muscles, but peak pressures cannot be sustained and only act for a second or two. It is therefore important to ensure that a lift will be a clean one, and that you will not be stuck half way, unable to bring the load up or down.

Most bending or lifting strains occur when inadequate preparation has gone into the task. Think before you lift. Is it

Lifting

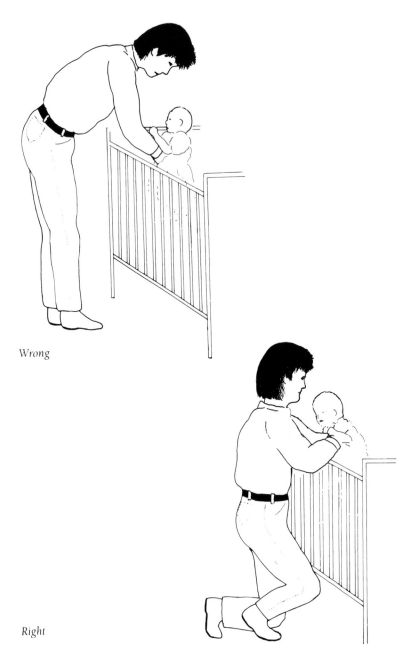

Wrong

Right

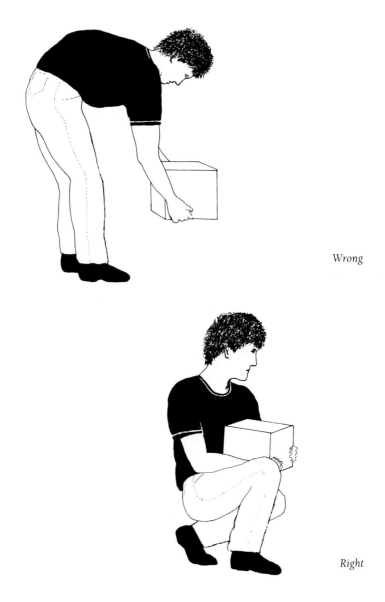

Wrong

Right

However precious your load, always ensure you hold it close to your body, bend your knees, and keep your back straight

Standing

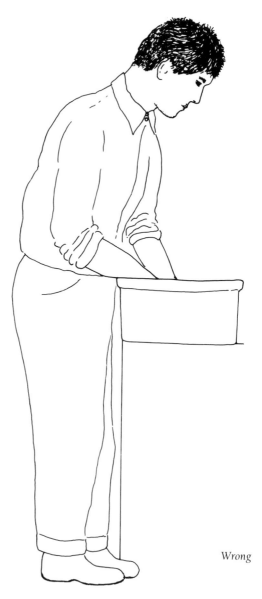

Wrong

When standing keep your back straight and avoid stooping. Carry your weight evenly on both legs. If waiting in a queue avoid rounded shoulders by adding a few inches to your height and 'standing tall'. When you walk, 'walk tall' and allow the arms to swing gently. Hands in pockets discourage good posture

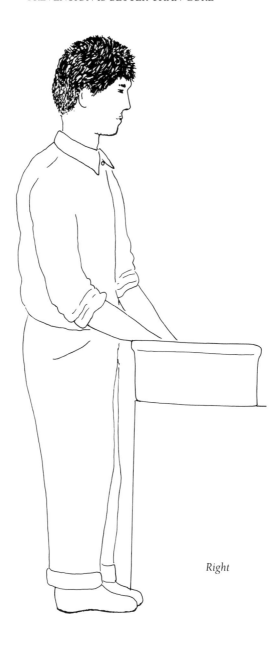

Right

really necessary? Ensure that your clothing is loose and is not going to constrict your movement. A tight belt may help to increase abdominal pressure. Ensure that you are standing on an even non-slip ground, free of obstructions. If you are lifting with assistance ensure that you both co-ordinate the movement together, and that your partner has a similar build so that neither one of you is subjected to overloading during the lift.

If you can share a load equally, divide it between the left and right hands. One heavy suitcase will pull you down on one side, making you swing your pelvis and lower back to compensate. Two smaller suitcases carried either side require less energy and subject you to significantly less strain.

CARE AT WORK

Employers who refer their staff for chiropractic treatment have found that it not only dramatically cuts absenteeism from back pain but that it raises working morale. Preliminary studies at the Taunton Cider Company in Somerset over a five year period have shown massive economic savings as a result of chiropractic care, and a major research project is shortly to begin with the employees of a division of British Gas.

In addition to caring for injured workers with chiropractic treatment many employers are now paying more attention to the working environment, and to measures that improve safety, comfort, and concentration. Although this may initially involve some degree of capital expenditure and changes to existing work practices, efficiency, increased output, and raised profits follow. Inadequate working conditions cause employees to waste energy and tire rapidly, increasing the likelihood of accidents, faulty workmanship, lost production, and joint or muscle strain. Back pain is second only to bronchitis as the major cause of days off work, and can be greatly reduced if expert advice is sought. Attention to ergonomics will increase production, raise its quality, and improve employee morale.

The chiropractor will assess tasks to be performed, weights to be lifted, equipment to be operated, and clothing to be worn. He or she will need to examine hoists and lifting aids, and learn the level of safety training and advice given to workers. Work surfaces will be recommended for minimizing postural fatigue for the sitting or standing employee. Some tasks suit those of a certain physique, and advice may be given on choosing the best person for the job. A selection of tasks which keep the worker mobile is preferable to one or two repetitive movements, and efficiency can often be improved by designing new working routines and repositioning work surfaces and equipment.

Efficiency and alertness in the office can be improved by advising on desk and chair heights, and by correctly positioning equipment such as word processors, visual display units, filing systems, and telephones. Secretaries often adopt bad habits in their teens, habitually placing copy material on the same side of the typewriter, thereby inducing neck and shoulder distortion. The filing cabinet you reach for behind your chair, or the telephone you tuck between chin and shoulder, may be examples of some of the habits you repeat countless times throughout the day, leading to ligament strain, muscle fatigue, and in time to degenerative arthritis. Contrary to popular belief, a number of studies, including those undertaken at the Taunton Cider Company, have shown that office workers are more vulnerable to back pain than manual workers.

Housework also brings problems. Working surfaces are often too low or too high. Too much time is spent partially bent forward over an ironing board or vacuum cleaner. Cupboards or clothes-lines set too high can cause overreaching strains that are as serious as bending strains. It is better to kneel to make a bed or to change a baby's nappy than to bend, but if bending is unavoidable remember to avoid holding the stooped or semi-stooped position for more than 15 seconds at a time. If you are forced to stand still for a long time, as when ironing a mountain of clothing, it is sometimes helpful to find a small footstool and to rest one leg at a time. If you choose this method it is essential you alternate sides every few minutes to avoid overloading the pelvis and lumbar spine on the weight bearing side.

Gardening brings its delights but also its torments. Before you set out be sure to warm yourself up with a few muscle stretching exercises, but avoid getting hot, as sweat in the small of the back can easily chill in a cold wind. At the outset plan how you will spend the next few hours. Avoid the temptation of spending too long at the same task. Select three jobs that require different physical activity, for example mowing, weeding, and digging. Allot 20 minutes in every hour to each task. In the same way that your garden increases yields and resists disease when proper crop rotation is observed, so your back increases production and resists strain with proper task rotation.

Choose tools which minimize bending or reaching, such as long-handled hoes, forks, rakes, and pruning shears. Avoid machines which must be dragged sideways at the end of a run. It is better to take two manageable loads on a wheel barrow than one large one that risks a twisting strain at the destination. Do not bend when you can kneel, and buy yourself kneeling pads or a low kneeling stool for the purpose. Avoid sudden pulling movements and use the correct tools, so that when removing tree roots you do not wrench away at them but dig and cut them out properly.

When digging, choose a long-handled spade so you can keep the hands further apart for improved leverage, and lift with the knees keeping the back straight. Stop and stretch often, but try not to arch the back whilst doing so. Always face your work squarely, and avoid working from the side with the trunk twisted. Do not overreach, but work as close to the job as is comfortable.

When you have finished gardening avoid slumping in a re-clining chair or bath for too long, and make sure you give your lumbar spine the proper support when you relax. Many problems are compounded by overstretching warm and well-worked ligaments in a slouched position at the day's end.

Specific occupations bring their specific types of strain. Some musicians are particularly at risk, and 'violinist's neck' and 'cellist's back' are well known to chiropractors. Chiropractors themselves often forget and work predominantly on one side of the treatment couch, as do dentists, thereby developing occupational distortions. Plumbers and electricians squeeze into low and inaccessible spaces, straining the neck or low back. Motor mechanics habitually bend over engines and gear-boxes. Indeed, every occupation, whether physically active or sedentary, brings its own potential spinal problem, because so much of our life is spent at work. Even spending the day in front of the television or reading a book may be storing up trouble. The secret is to vary routine, frequently change position, avoid sitting or standing still for more than half an hour at a time, and to walk for short distances every hour.

POSTURE AND PREGNANCY

During pregnancy a number of hormonal changes occur which allow the ligaments of the pelvis to expand during childbirth. However, they also cause all the body's ligaments to stretch when subjected to strain. As the purpose of ligaments is to prevent a joint from overreaching, joint damage in the lumbar spine is a frequent occurrence, especially during the middle and late stages when the enlarging abdomen starts to shift the centre of gravity behind the weight-bearing lumbar discs. It is important that the lumbar spine and pelvis are monitored by a chiropractor during and after pregnancy so that corrections can be made that will minimize back strain, improve muscle tone, and aid the delivery of the baby.

A mother is particularly vulnerable in the first 6 months after giving birth, as the ligament-relaxing hormone Relaxin may remain in the body that long. Care must be taken to avoid partial or full bending, especially if this is to be sustained. Lifting and carrying the baby, its crib, and all the paraphernalia associated with it must call for extra care, especially when getting in and out of cars. Changing nappies, bathing the infant, and lifting it in and out of its cot all involve risk. Minimize stooping by using higher tables, or kneel where possible. Hold weights close to your body and face the task in hand to avoid twisting. Try to share heavier loads with partners, relatives, or friends. During this stage not only should you ask your chiropractor to check your own back, but also take this ideal opportunity for a spinal check on your new baby, so that problems acquired during the birth can be identified and corrected when they are easiest to treat, before the baby begins weight bearing.

TELL-TALE SIGNS

It is important that you become aware of those tell-tale signs that give you advance warning of impending spinal problems. An ache or pain is usually the first warning you will receive, and at times it may be accompanied by muscle spasm. If the symptoms can clearly be related to a known cause and they clear within 24 hours all you may need to do is avoid repeating the provoking factor. If pain lasts longer or symptoms recur regularly then you probably have a malfunctioning spinal or pelvic joint. This malfunction can bring on an overload elsewhere in the spine and trouble will arise when you perform certain movements or adopt certain waking or sleeping positions. It is time to seek the care and advice of a qualified chiropractor.

There are other signs which should prompt you to seek professional advice. Pain or discomfort on coughing, sneezing, or passing a bowel motion may be warning you of a disc problem. Headaches, dizziness, vertigo, ringing in the ears (tinnitus), or visual disturbances can indicate a neck condition, as can scalp, throat, or facial pain. Breathing difficulties and chest tightness may also mask a spinal problem. Crackling and crunching in the joints (crepitus) may be a sign of early wear and tear, and although osteoarthritic degenerative changes are as normal to the ageing process as wrinkles on the face, it is wise to check with a qualified chiropractor the moment any discomfort is felt. Undue restriction can then be cleared and premature degeneration of any one overloaded joint reduced.

Tingling or numbness may result from sitting or sleeping awkwardly, and goes when the faulty position is corrected. If it becomes a regular occurrence it is likely you are suffering nerve interference at a spinal level. Muscle weakness is another symptom of nerve interference, so that grip strength is lost, cutlery is accidentally dropped, climbing up or down stairs rapidly tires the muscles, or standing on tiptoes becomes difficult. Co-ordination may also be impaired when spinal nerves fail to function properly.

Sometimes joint restriction comes on almost imperceptibly. You realize that you must turn your body to reverse the car as neck movement is no longer sufficient on its own. In the morning it is a struggle to put on shoes or socks, and you can no longer slide on your jacket or cardigan with ease. Combing your hair or reaching behind to do up a brassiere is no longer easy. As you get out of bed to walk to the bathroom you feel the stiffness which needs several minutes of stretching to overcome. Stiffness as you get out of the car or a chair may also warn you during the day. These are all signs that your joints are becoming restricted and need the attention of a qualified chiropractor to restore range of movement.

ACTION IN INJURY

If sharp joint pain or muscle spasm suddenly strikes, it is important you know how to minimize damage. Do not reach for a heat pad or soak in a hot bath. Instead make yourself an ice-pack and place it over the injured area. A packet of peas or sweetcorn from the freezer is ideal as it can be moulded into shape. If your low back is at fault lie comfortably on your side or back with your knees drawn up to relieve pressure.

If the problem is with your neck lie on your back or side with a rolled up towel supporting the neck (but not the head). With a thin cloth wrapped around the ice pack to prevent skin adhesion place it directly against the site of injury. It will be uncomfortable at first, but leave it in place for 15 to 20 minutes. During this time the inflammatory process will be slowed down considerably and can often be bypassed. This will speed recovery, provided the area is rested. The ice-pack should be repeated every couple of hours until the inflammation has subsided, whereupon gentle movements should be attempted if painless.

Vulnerable joints should be stabilized, and it may be necessary to immobilize the neck with a coiled towel or soft collar and the low back with a tight belt or corset. Supports should never be relied upon for more than a few days, as they detract from one's own muscle tone, but in the short term they can reduce the risk of further strain whilst protecting the area from painful and harmful relapses during critical early recovery stages. Avoid stairs, rough ground, lifting or jarring movements, and deep chairs. Avoid twisting of any kind, and take special care getting in and out of bed and cars.

It is important you consult a qualified chiropractor as soon as possible for diagnosis of the problem and for management of the recovery period. The chiropractor will advise on ice-packs, heat, support, rest, and exercise for your particular problem. He or she will tell you when to increase your activity and how you can best speed recovery at home. You should resist the advice of well-meaning amateurs who may not appreciate that identical symptoms do not necessarily arise from identical problems, but require individual assessment and professional handling.

Once faulty joint movement is identified, chiropractic adjustment of joints, muscles, or soft tissues will bring about a speedy recovery and early return to work, whilst reducing the risk of recurrence. Even if symptoms subside on their own without treatment, so long as hidden malfunction persists the likelihood of a more serious relapse is increased. Spinal corrections by a trained chiropractor will restore joint function and minimize the risk of further attacks.

Chapter 5

SPECIFIC EXERCISES

Sages do not treat those who are already ill; they rather instruct those who are not yet ill . . . The superior physician helps before the early budding of disease. The inferior physician begins to help when the disease has already developed. *Huang Ti* (Twenty-Seventh Century BC)

More than four out of five people will experience a spell of debilitating back or neck pain during their lifetime. Usually they are warned before it happens — with a sense of weakness or insecurity in the spine. Attacks can often be warded off by improving mobility and by toning muscles. A periodic check-up by a chiropractor to ensure that joints are moving correctly is important, but in the meantime many problems can be averted or kept at bay by specific exercises.

Although the symptoms may be identical to those of friends, neighbours, or colleagues, there are many different causes of spinal malfunction that may produce similar symptoms. An exercise that suits one person may not be right for another, even though they may be experiencing the same pain in the same place. Even some of the more popular exercises may not be suitable for you, and the first part of this chapter will direct you to 'universal exercises' which can be performed by almost all patients with the minimum of risk.

Chiropractors are equipped as experts in spinal care, and your chiropractor will direct you to the most appropriate exercises for your own back. Some of the more common ones are described under the headings that follow the universal exercises, but they should not be performed until you have been examined.

UNIVERSAL EXERCISES

Many of the patients encountered by chiropractors are suffering from problems brought on by alteration to the normal curves of the spine. As the facet joints at the back of the spine are highly pain-sensitive, the action of cramming them together or holding them open in a fully gapped state can rapidly induce pain, and all exercises must be designed to avoid either extreme. Toe-touching exercises are particularly dangerous, especially from the standing position, when body weight not only stresses gapped lumbar facets but overloads the discs as well, and these should be avoided even when lying down. Leg raising exercises tend to overload the lumbar area, for as the legs are lifted from the floor the lumbar curve is exaggerated under the load of the lower limbs.

Both overweight and weak abdominal muscles allow the abdomen to drift forward, cramming together the lower lumbar facet joints inducing a sway-back posture. This posture can be exaggerated by the wearing of high heeled shoes, and women are particularly susceptible. Such an action will not only increase the lower lumbar curve, but is met by a compensatory increase higher up in both the thoracic and cervical curves. This postural state probably complicates more than half the cases met by chiropractors.

At the other end of the scale, children are often taught to adopt the military stance, driving the shoulders back to eliminate the natural thoracic curve. This not only crams together the facet joints of the upper thoracic area but it puts strain on neck muscles and irritates the vulnerable area between the lower thoracic and upper lumbar spine.

We are often told to mobilize the neck by rotating or rolling back the head to extremes of left and right. This will probably be harmless if our neck is in pristine condition, but it is quite common for the atlas vertebra to be rotated slightly forward, either to the right or left. Rotation or head rolling should never be induced towards the side of such a forward displacement and, even in the absence of an atlas distortion, common degenerative changes in the neck can be further complicated by stressful rotary movements.

The following have been named 'universal exercises', not because they can be guaranteed to benefit every patient, but because they should not aggravate underlying problems and can be performed safely by almost everybody if carried out correctly. Many other exercises are excellent for the purpose for which they were designed, but they often run the risk of causing strain if fairly common postural or joint deficiencies are present.

These universal exercises are devised to free the pelvic, lumbar, thoracic and cervical areas with the minimum of strain, and an all-important abdominal muscle exercise is added. It is essential that all exercises are carefully and correctly applied, and in the event of any pain they should be stopped immediately and not resumed until you have consulted your chiropractor. To be fully effective these universal exercises should be performed slowly, smoothly and carefully, with each exercise repeated 20 times twice daily.

FOR THE PELVIS

This has been called the backward cycle exercise because it resembles a reversed bicycling motion as the sacro-iliac joint is carried through its full range of movement. It is important that you remember to retain your normal lumbar curve throughout, that you do not stoop in any direction, and that you keep yourself firmly in the standing position. Although the composite parts have been subdivided for ease of comprehension, the whole exercise should be performed in one slow smooth cycling action.

1. Standing, with one hand firmly gripping a piece of heavy furniture for stabilization, slowly raise your right leg in front of you. When the muscles at the back of your leg tighten bend the knee, bringing the heel towards the buttock as your thigh is raised into the horizontal position.

2. Push the heel straight back behind you, keeping it high off the ground until the knee is almost straightened behind you.

3. As the knee straightens bring the leg downward so that you end in the starting position.

4. Still steadying yourself with the same hand, repeat the cycle with the left leg to complete your first set.

5. Continue until you have completed 20 sets.

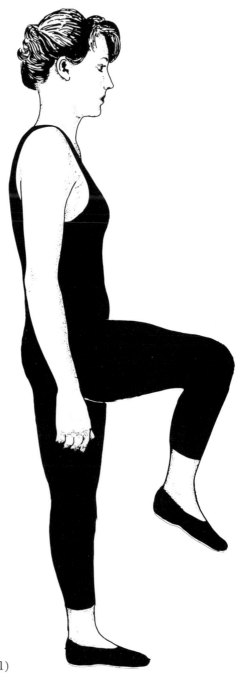

Backward cycle (1)

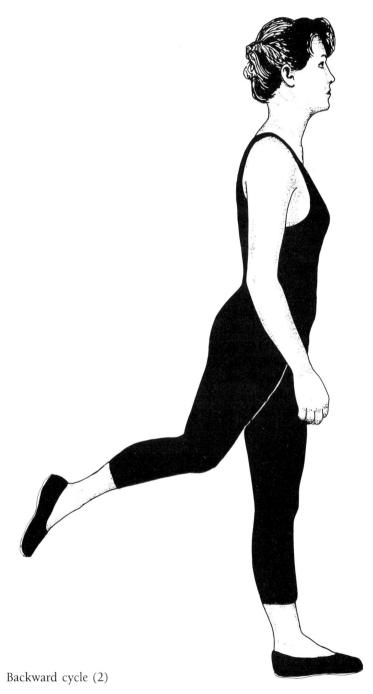

Backward cycle (2)

FOR THE LUMBAR SPINE

Find a piece of furniture that you can straddle with your thighs to prevent you from shifting to the right and left as you bend your lumbar spine sideways. A table corner is ideal as you can grip the sides with your thighs, standing with your feet apart and in line with your shoulders. If you point the toes about 30–40 degrees inward you will stretch the piriformis muscle as you bend sideways, and this is beneficial in a number of low back conditions. During the exercise ensure that you drift neither forward nor backward, as it is important you do not compromise the facet joints when you bend to the side.

1. With your arms hanging loosely beside you and in this stable position astride the table corner, slowly bend your lumbar spine to one side as far as you can comfortably go.

2. When this point has been reached slowly straighten the spine until you reach the starting position again.

3. Repeat the side bend to the other side to complete your first set.

4. As with the previous exercise all movements should be undertaken slowly in one continuous smooth cycle, until 20 sets have been completed.

FOR THE THORACIC SPINE

It is difficult to bend the thoracic spine backward and forward without increasing and decreasing the natural neck and low-back curves at the same time. During this exercise allow the neck and back to go along for the ride, but do not consciously carry them forward or backward. Allow gravity and your normal posture to keep the head and low back in natural equilibrium. In spite of this advice you may be surprised to learn that you start the exercise sitting with the thoracic spine in a fully slumped position.

1. Sitting on a stool or on the edge of a bed, allow your thoracic spine to slump into the forward position with your shoulders naturally rolling forward as your shoulder muscles fully relax and your arms hang limply beside you. It is important you retain the low-back and neck curves, so do not let the lumbar

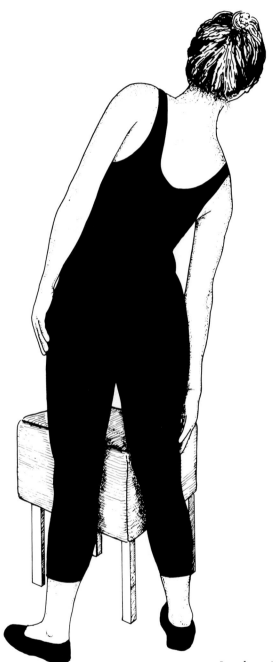

Lumbar side stretch

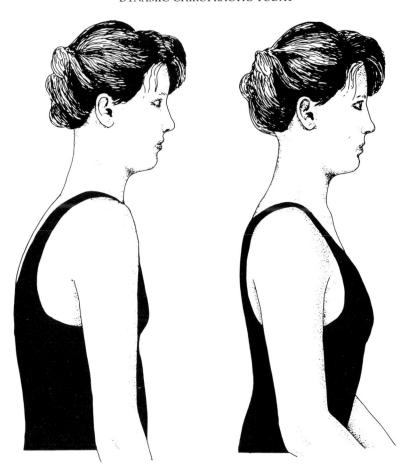

Sitting thoracic extension

    spine slump and fix your eyes on an object straight in front of you.

2.   Slowly straighten the thoracic spine up and out of the slumped position. Do not do this at the expense of arching the lumbar spine, as this could cram and irritate lumbar facet joints. Do not draw your shoulders back into the military position, but keep them fully relaxed throughout this exercise. Ensure the head does not roll backward by keeping your eyes fixed in front of you.

3.   When you have straightened the thoracic spine as far as it will comfortably go reverse the process so that you return to

the slumped position and complete your first set.

4. Repeat the cycle 20 times, remembering to protect the low-back and neck curves throughout, and ensuring that the shoulders remain in a forward relaxed position to protect the thoracic spine. Although the exercise may seem very simple it is difficult to remember all the commandments at first, and you should remain conscious of the 'do nots' until the exercise has become second nature to you.

FOR THE NECK

This has been called the rainbow exercise because the eyes are fixed on an imaginary rainbow directly in front of you. Imagine the scene. Turn your head to look straight at the lower left hand side of the rainbow as it fades into the horizon ahead of you. Slowly follow the bow upward to its bright apex in the sky. Continue from left to right as you follow the rainbow down to earth again, far away on the horizon. At this stage allow the head to drop down in search of the pot of gold. Reverse the cycle from right to left to complete one set, and perform 20 sets in all. To lock the thoracic spine keep the arms crossed throughout.

It may seem rather fanciful to conjure up a rainbow every time you perform this exercise. However, there are very sound reasons behind it. A rainbow starts on the horizon and not at your feet, so your head does not drop down until the movement has been completed. As you follow the bow upward your head is carried through an angle of no more than 45 degrees. You will never find the rainbow directly above you, and you are therefore prevented from over-extending the head backward. When a rainbow lies straight in front of you its two pillars are not so far apart that you have to rotate to extremes of left and right to follow them. Full neck rotation to left or right must be strictly avoided in any universally safe exercise.

The aim is to carry your neck through a composite of movements that will exercise it without overreaching. Full neck rotation or extension backward must never ever be performed if you have any history of dizziness or have ever suffered a stroke, however mild. Care must also be taken if there are degenerative changes in your neck (arthritis, osteoarthrosis or spondylosis), as neck exercises carried to any of the extremes can very easily trigger an attack of acute pain and inflammation in such cases. Your imaginary rainbow may never lead you to that pot of gold, but it will ensure you a safe journey if you perform the exercise correctly.

FOR THE ABDOMINAL MUSCLES

About nine out of ten adults have less than ideal abdominal muscle tone and will benefit from straightening these muscles. Abdominal muscles are weakened by physical inactivity, abdominal operations, overweight, and pregnancy, and the resulting postural changes shift the body's centre of gravity so that lower lumbar vertebrae risk overload.

When we use our bodies to lift or bend, much of the strain is taken by tightening the abdominal muscles, raising pressure within the abdominal cavity. This works like the pressure in a motorcar tyre, when tonnes of weight can be borne and carried only when the tyre is inflated. When the air is released the tyre wall collapses. When weak abdominal muscles reduce our capacity to generate much pressure the wall of the abdomen offers little resistance and the lumbar spine is left to take the full burden. The following exercise is therefore a very important one.

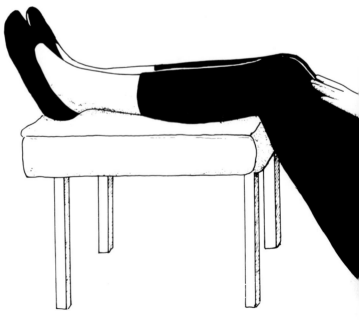

1. Lie on your back with your hips and knees bent and your lower legs resting on a chair. Ensure that you place a small rolled up towel or a small cushion in the arch of the back to preserve the normal lumbar curve throughout this exercise. Place a support under your neck but not under your head.

2. From this position raise the shoulders 3–4 inches (7–10 cm) off the floor, but do not flex the head fully forward as you do so. Hold this position for a count of five.

3. Slowly lower the shoulders to the starting position and allow yourself to recover before repeating. Start with ten repetitions, gradually increasing to 20.

If you feel discomfort in your neck and need to support it whilst the head is raised off the ground, clasp your fingers behind your lower neck. Make sure that you preserve the neck curve and do not force the head forward.

MOBILIZING EXERCISES FOR THE BACK AND PELVIS

None of these exercises should be performed until you have the approval of your chiropractor.

Shoulder raise

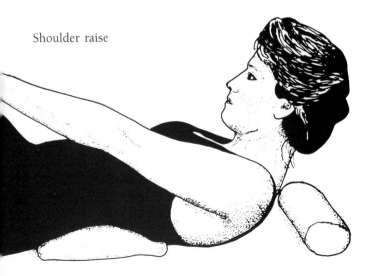

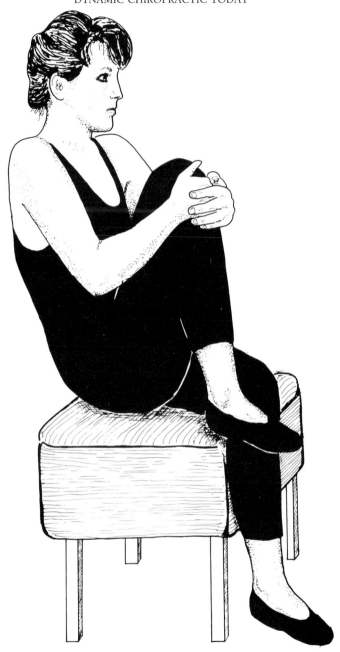

Sacro-iliac stretch

SACRO-ILIAC STRETCH

This is a gentle and effortless exercise and is performed sitting down.

1. Sit with the thighs fully supported by the bed, stool, bench, chair or table.

2. Slowly draw your right knee towards your chest, keeping the back straight, and hold it there at full stretch for a count of five. Repeat with the other knee. For maximum sacro-iliac stretching draw the knee towards the opposite shoulder and hold for five. Try not to let your spine bow backward and keep your head level.

A stiff sacro-iliac joint causes the lumbar spine to take on loads normally absorbed by the elastic ligaments of these joints. Therefore this exercise is best done as you get out of bed and before you set out on chores which may otherwise stress the back.

Repeat ten times, and any time later in the day when you have been sitting for a while.

LUMBAR SIDE BENDS

It is difficult to improve on the exercise for the low back in the universal exercise section. The stabilizing table corner can be dispensed with provided care is taken to bend from the lumbar spine and to avoid any side sway.

THE CAT STRETCH

Those who have observed a cat arising from its slumbers will have watched the way it stretches its spine before stepping out. This is also a useful exercise for humans as they get out of bed.

1. Kneel forward with your hips bent, arms straight, and hands on the floor.

2. Arch your back upward to the ceiling as fully as it will go, whilst lowering your head.

3. Raise your head as you lower your spine into a deep 'U' curve. Repeat this exercise five times.

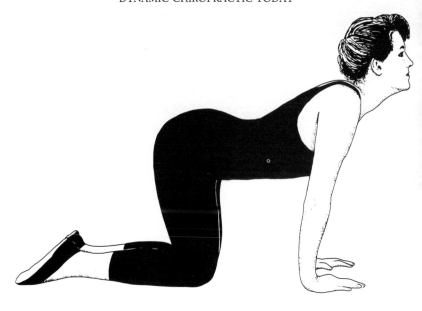

Cat stretch (1)

THE HIP STRETCH

One of the first signs of arthritis in the ball and socket joint of the hip is restriction. If this starts to occur, mobility must be maintained to prevent further degeneration.

1. Lie on your back with your left leg straight. The right leg is bent at the knee which is flared out to the side as the ankle is positioned to rest just above the left knee cap. Place the right hand against the right thigh.

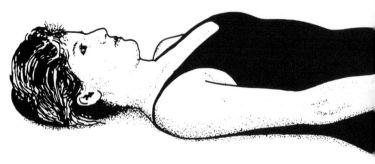

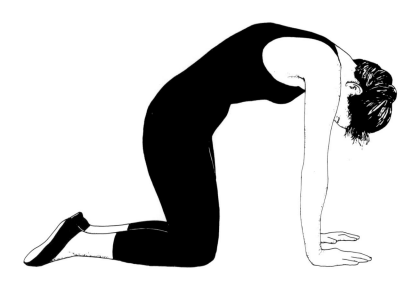

Cat stretch (2)

2. Force the knee away from the mid line and towards the floor, assisting with the right hand if necessary. Hold for a count of five. Repeat with the left leg and perform five sets.

If your hip is very tight you may feel some pain in the groin on forcing the hip outwards. This is the only exercise listed here where the exercise should be performed right into the pain barrier, but be certain to discuss it with your chiropractor first. Try to avoid stressing the knee joint as you push the leg to its limit.

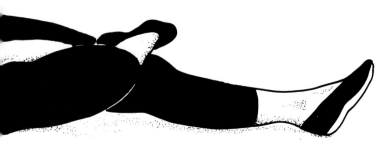

Hip stretch

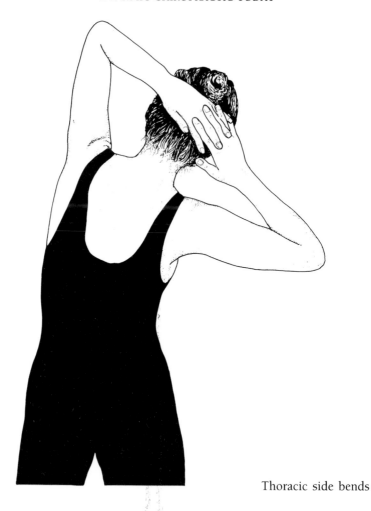

Thoracic side bends

THORACIC SIDE BENDS

Although the ribs naturally limit spinal movement in the thorax it is important to maintain mobility.

1. Stand with your feet apart and your hands behind your head.

2. Lean to the right as if to point the right elbow to the floor and the left to the ceiling. Hold for a count of five before returning to the neutral position. Repeat to the left and perform five sets. Take care to move from the upper back and not from the lumbar spine.

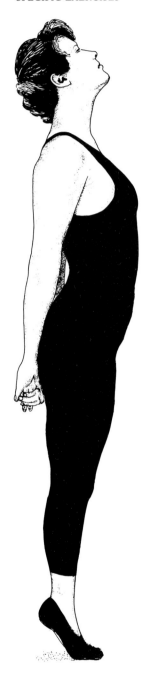

Thoracic extension

THORACIC EXTENSION

Because of the position of the upper ribs spinal extension is not easily achieved in this region. This must never be performed by a patient with a military stance.

1. Stand with your feet apart and your hands clasped behind your back with elbows straight.

2. Breathe in and pull downwards with the arms, whilst standing on tiptoe and tilting your head backward. Patients with a sway back should avoid the tiptoe stance and the head tilt. Repeat five times.

SHOULDER ROTATION

This exercise loosens the shoulders and upper back.

1. Stand with your feet apart and your hands clasped behind your back with the elbows relaxed. Draw the shoulders up high.

2. Rotate the shoulders first backward and then forward. This exercise should be avoided in many lower neck conditions. Repeat ten times.

NECK MOBILIZING EXERCISES

None of these exercises should be performed until you have the approval of your chiropractor. Some neck mobilizing exercises can bring about a dizzy light-headed feeling at times, and if this occurs you must stop the exercise immediately and not resume it until you have consulted your chiropractor. Pain is another indicator that should not be ignored, and you should avoid any neck exercise that provokes pain until the inflammation has subsided.

GENERAL NECK MOBILIZATION

This is a composite of three neck exercises done sitting or standing, and as your chiropractor may wish you to emphasize individual elements, each is described separately.

1. Flexion-Extension

Bend your head forward, attempting to bring your chin towards your Adam's apple. Then gently reverse the procedure, extending the head backward as far as it will comfortably go. Repeat before moving on to the next element.

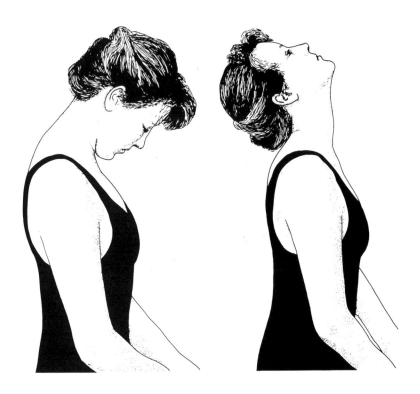

Neck flexion-extension

2. Side Bending

Do not turn the head into rotation but gently tilt the head as far as it will go to the right, as if to press the ear to the shoulder. When a comfortable extreme has been reached reverse the movement, tilting the head to the left. Repeat before moving to the next element.

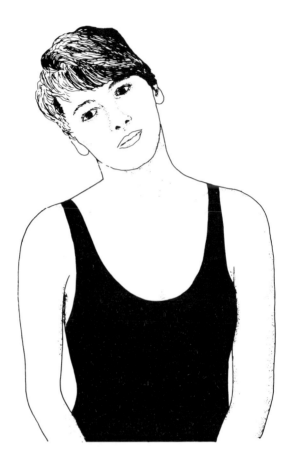

Neck side bends

3. Rotation

Keeping your shoulders down, carefully turn your head to the right as if to look over your right shoulder. When the maximum range of rotation has been reached hold for a count of five before reversing to look over your left shoulder and hold. Repeat.

These three elements should be repeated five times, although your chiropractor may wish you to increase or decrease repetitions of one or two of the elements.

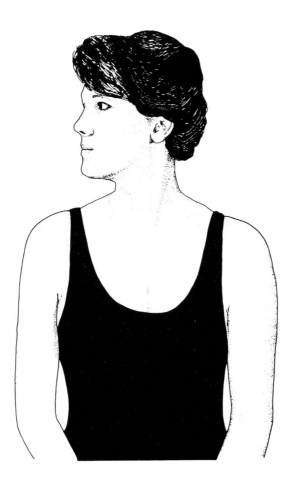

Neck rotation

THE CHICKEN WALK EXERCISE

The joint between the base of the skull and the top of the spine may need specific exercise. If you have ever watched a chicken walk you may have observed its head remaining horizontal whilst being carried forward and backward with each stride. This horizontal carriage is the essential element of the exercise, lending its name most descriptively.

105

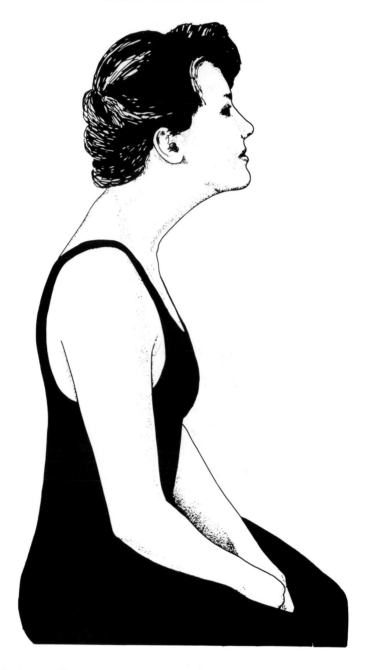

Chicken walk (1)

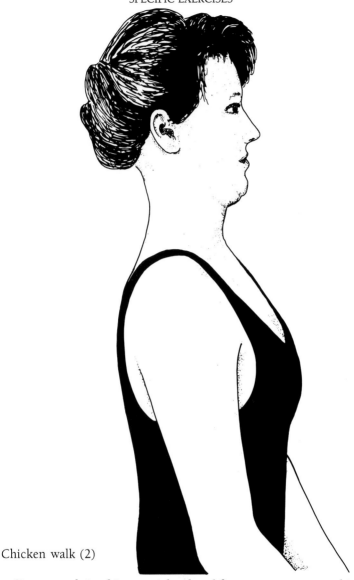

Chicken walk (2)

Sit or stand. Looking straight ahead fix your eyes on an object. Steadily keeping your eyes on that point, push your head forward, keeping the chin up. When the full range of movement has been reached push the head back as far as it will go, but this time tucking the chin well in. Keep the eyes level at all times and do not look down or up as you exercise.

Repeat five times.

MUSCLE STRENGTHENING
EXERCISES FOR THE BACK

Muscle weakness will frequently allow joints to become overloaded, bringing about pain and swelling. Weak postural muscles cause ligaments to lengthen and joints to dangerously overreach. Isometric exercises are often the most effective way of building up strength. During these exercises you should breathe normally and try to avoid holding your breath.

Many postural problems arise because weak abdominal muscles allow the abdomen to drift forward, increasing the lumbar curve beyond its natural capacity. If all other muscles are forgotten, the ones that cannot be ignored are the abdominals.

As with all the exercises not in the universal section, your chiropractor's advice should be sought before embarking on any of these. If in any doubt do the abdominal exercise in the universal section, which is just as effective as the following more popular versions.

UPPER ABDOMINALS

1. Lie on your back with your knees bent, feet flat on the floor.

Upper abdominals

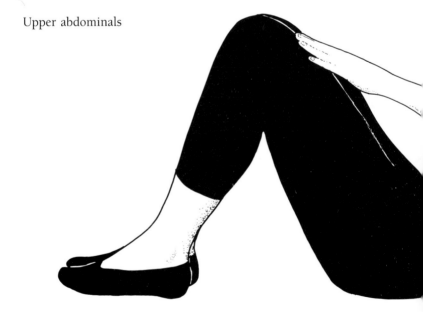

2. Slowly curl the head and shoulders up while moving your straightened arms to touch your knees. Hold for a count of five, and gently relax back. Repeat five times, but gradually build up to fifteen repetitions over several months. Do not worry if you cannot raise your shoulders off the ground at first. Tensing the muscles and holding them tight will start the process, and within weeks or months you should be able to reach the required position. This emphasizes fibres of the upper abdominal muscles.

LOWER ABDOMINALS

1. Lie on your back with the knees bent, feet flat on the floor.

2. Straighten the right leg so that it is extended to about 45 degrees from the floor. Straighten the left leg, but lower it so that the heel is about 4 inches (10 cm) from the floor.

3. Alternate the two legs slowly so that as the right leg lowers the left one rises. It is important you do not allow the back to slip into extension. Repeat five times, building up to 15 repetitions in the coming months. This emphasizes the lower abdominal muscle fibres, but take great care to discontinue if discomfort is felt.

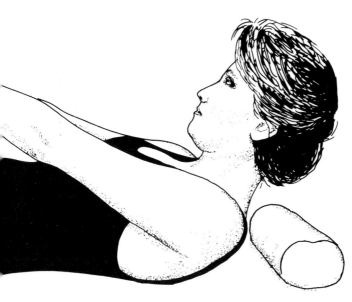

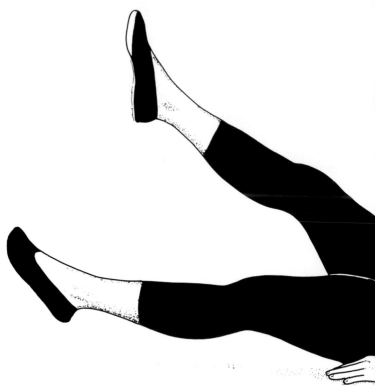

In cases of sway back this exercise should be avoided altogether. Less serious cases may sometimes benefit by modifying the upper abdominal position, so that the legs are crossed over, when a held sit-up will exercise more lower-abdominal muscle fibres. In this instance the feet should be stabilized by your partner or placed under some heavy item of furniture.

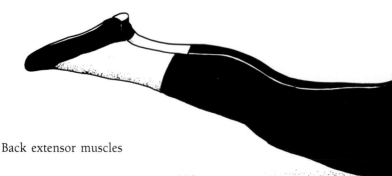

Back extensor muscles

Lower abdominals

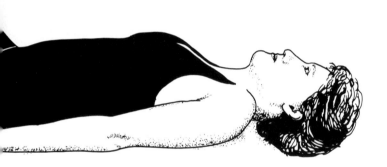

BACK EXTENSOR MUSCLES

Although strong abdominal muscles provide the key to a healthy back it is important that the paraspinal muscles running along the length of the spine are well toned. Care should be taken with

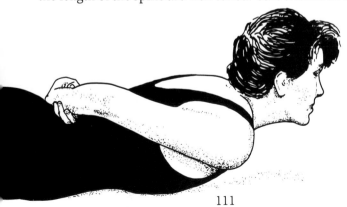

back extension exercises, which can irritate already inflamed spinal joints, so that at the first sign of discomfort (as with any of these exercises) you must stop until you have discussed the symptoms with your chiropractor.

1. Lie on your front with your hands linked together behind you.

2. Slowly raise your head, shoulders, and straightened legs from the floor and hold for a count of five. Rest for a count of ten before repeating. Start with five repetitions, building up slowly to ten.

HIP MUSCLES

A number of important spinal muscles are attached to the hips and pelvis, and a strong foundation is therefore important for stability. An exercise to strengthen the outer hip muscles is frequently prescribed.

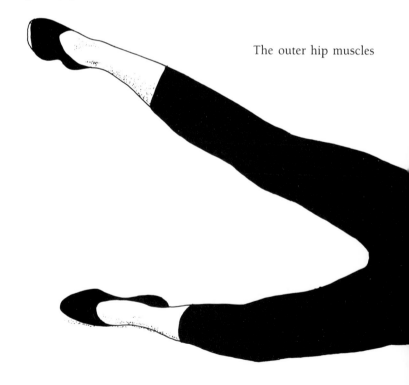

The outer hip muscles

1. Lie on your left side with your head on a pillow or with your arm tucked up as a support. Bend your left leg to provide stability.

2. Raise your straightened right leg as far as it will go and hold for a count of five. Repeat five times. Turn over and repeat the exercise, raising the left leg.

MUSCLE STRENGTHENING EXERCISES FOR THE NECK

As with the back, isometric exercises to strengthen the neck should be accompanied by normal even breathing, and holding the breath should be avoided. These exercises follow the three elements shown in the section on neck mobilizing, but here movement is prevented as the muscles tense against resistance. Five repetitions are recommended, later building up to ten, but your chiropractor may advise you to start with only one or two in your special circumstances, or if your neck muscles are very weak. You must never be tempted to increase repetitions if any discomfort is felt.

FLEXION-EXTENSION

1. Flexion: Bringing your hands to your forehead, push your head downward against their resistance. Hold for a count of

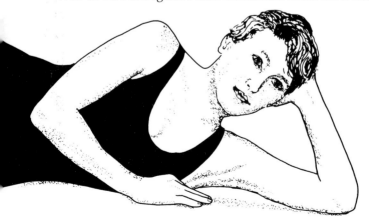

five, and then slowly relax. Repeat before moving to extension.

2. Extension: Bring your hands behind your head and interlock your fingers. Push your head back against their resistance. Hold for a count of five and slowly relax. Repeat before moving to the next exercise..

SIDE BENDING

Bring your arms up and cup the palms of your hands over your ears, fingers pointing outwards. Press your head to the right as if to touch the ear to the shoulder, but as with all these isometric exercises, no movement should occur as your hands resist the pressure. Hold for a count of five and slowly relax. Repeat to the left before moving to the next exercise.

ROTATION

Bring your arms up and cup the palms of your hands over your ears, fingers pointing forward over the forehead with thumbs behind the ears. Attempt against resistance to look over your right shoulder. Hold for a count of five and slowly relax. Repeat to the left.

MUSCLE STRETCHING EXERCISES

It is frequently found that back pain sufferers not only need to loosen their pelvis and spine but also need to stretch tight muscles which may have brought on back strain directly, or be hindering recovery.

HAMSTRINGS

Tight hamstrings will produce a pulling sensation in the back of your thighs as you bend at your hips towards the floor with your back and legs held straight. These muscles are attached to the pelvis and can impair its mobility if they are excessively taut.

1. Sit lengthways along the left side of a firm bed, bench, or

table; your right leg should be stretched out on the surface while the left overhangs, bent at the knee, with the foot on the floor.

2. Reach forward with your hands as if to touch your right foot, but do not force yourself into pain. Hold for a count of five, and then relax back. Repeat the stretch five times before changing position to stretch the left leg.

ILIO-PSOAS MUSCLE

The psoas muscles pass from upper lumbar vertebrae to the upper thigh and are joined by the iliac muscles from the pelvis. An excessively tight ilio-psoas muscle impairs hip, pelvis, and spinal movement. It has also been implicated in a number of conditions beyond back pain, such as headaches, dizziness, asthma, and lack of energy.

The hamstrings

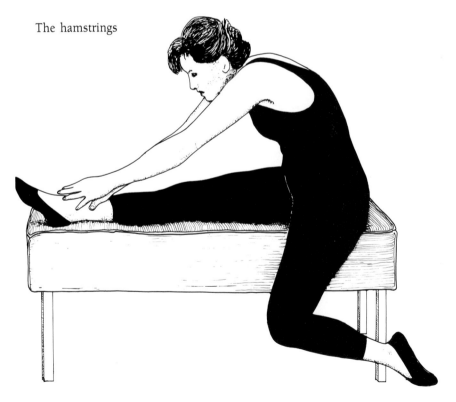

Ilio-psoas muscle

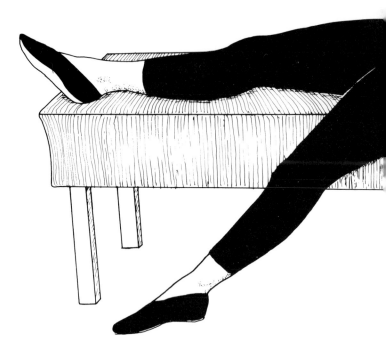

1. Lie back lengthways along the left side of a firm bed, bench, or table, with the right leg stretched out along the surface, and the left overhanging.

2. Let the left leg relax and allow gravity to stretch the ilio-psoas

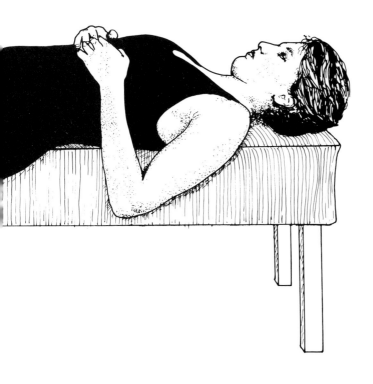

gently, using the leg's own weight to do so. Allow the leg to hang for a count of ten before changing position to stretch the right side. Repeat the set three times. Your chiropractor may instruct you to stretch one side only.

Chapter 6

HISTORIC ROOTS

And when you can, read the original descriptions of the masters who, with crude methods of study, saw so clearly. *Sir William Osler* (1849–1919)

CHIROPRACTIC'S ORIGINS

To understand why chiropractic has become the most successful form of complementary medicine in the Western world it is important to appreciate not only its recent history but also the circumstances which led to its establishment in the United States in 1895. Manipulation was by no means a novel therapy at the end of the nineteenth century, having been used extensively throughout history, yet its application as a separate system of natural medicine set it into headlong opposition with established medicine. The centuries leading up to the birth of chiropractic had seen conflicting philosophies of medicine develop from ancient theories, and whilst the new medical practice shut out concepts of holism from its craft, it was left to the chiropractor and others to re-espouse holistic principles. Examination of the manipulative approach and the evolution of medical thought within the history of healing will help to explain the development of chiropractic at a time when established concepts were being challenged and the world was ready to be turned upside down by the events of the twentieth century.

EARLY MANIPULATIVE THERAPY

Daniel David Palmer (1845–1913), styled the 'discoverer' of

chiropractic, looked on Aesculapius (1250 BC) and later Hippocrates (460 BC) as the founders of chiropractic concepts and practice. However, long before the Grecian civilization came into being physicians had manipulated patients in the Far East, as is recorded in Chinese writings of 2700 BC. The Egyptian *Papyrus of New York*, thought to belong to the eighteenth century before Christ, describes the use of manipulation for various neck injuries. There have even been claims that prehistoric cave paintings of the Aurignacian period uncovered during the construction of France's Paris to Cannes trans-subway system depict manipulation in progress nearly 20,000 years ago, but this interpretation of such a primitive and symbolic art form does risk entering the realms of fancy.

The earliest valid illustration of spinal manipulation is a fifth century BC votive relief sculpted in marble and excavated from the Aesculapian hospital in Piraeus, Greece. It clearly depicts the pre-Hippocratic healer Aesculapius as he manipulates the upper thoracic spine, and Palmer acknowledged that these methods now 'rediscovered and known as chiropractic were also known and practised by Aesculapius and his followers'.

HIPPOCRATES AND MANIPULATION

In looking to the ancient Greeks as originators of chiropractic philosophy, Palmer was undoubtedly recalling the words of the Master Physician, Hippocrates of Kos: 'It is most necessary to know the nature of the spine, what its natural purposes are, for such a knowledge will be requisite for many diseases.' Like Hippocrates, Palmer was critical of the established approach which he regarded as cruel and blinkered. Hippocrates had condemned the common practice of hanging a man upside down from a ladder to cure spinal problems, which he considered had been abused: 'It is disgraceful in any art, and especially in medicine, to make parade of much trouble, display, and talk, and then do no good.'

Palmer regarded surgery and drugs as too drastic an approach in the quest for healing at a time when some physicians were still cauterizing or applying leeches to the tender spinal area, and when the cure was often more damaging than the disease. Emulating his mentor he developed a humane system of care based not on tradition nor on ill-considered formulae but on the conscientious examination of the spine accompanied by gentle manipulative correction.

Hippocrates had set himself against the medical system of his day which was based upon the cult figure of Aesculapius, and which was founded not on observation and analysis but on various temple rites. Hippocrates challenged it with a method of careful diagnosis that not only looked at the symptoms themselves but regarded such aspects as hygiene, diet, environment, and climate with equal importance. Some 2,350 years later Palmer criticized a system which looked at 'disease' as a force to be conquered externally with drugs or the surgeon's knife. He held that physical injury, toxins, or the patient's psychological state accounted for disease, and that they could be corrected by mobilizing the body's innate mechanism of self-cure from within and not through external agencies.

Palmer acknowledged that the principles of chiropractic were 'founded upon the laws as old as the Greek prophet', but regarded himself as an innovator creating 'the art of adjusting vertebrae, using the spinous and transverse processes as levers'. Indeed, little had changed in the art of manipulation since the days of Hippocrates when the patient had been placed face down on a wooden bed whilst assistants stretched the spine by pulling the shoulders and hips apart:

> The physician, or an assistant who is strong and not untrained, should put the palm of his hand on the hump, and the palm of the other on that, to reduce it forcibly. . . . This reduction method is also very harmless; indeed, it will do no harm even if one sits on the hump while extension is applied, and makes succussion by raising himself; nay, there is nothing against putting one's foot on the hump, and making gentle succussion by bringing one's weight upon it.

These methods were recorded by the Hippocratic Corpus, scholar physicians of Alexandria who established the classical Greek traditions, which found their way into Roman medicine.

ROME AND CLAUDIUS GALEN

In common with many conquering civilizations the Romans absorbed from their vassals the very best aspects of their culture. From Greece they took art, learning, and medicine, importing

Greek physicians to tend the health of their new high-society. Indeed, the most famous of all Roman physicians, Claudius Galen, was born a Greek. Arriving in Rome in 162 AD he was later to claim 'whoever seeks fame need only become familiar with all I have achieved', and medicine was dominated by his influence for over 1,500 years. His herbal 'Galenicals' were extensively used in medicine until the last century, and his methods of Hippocratic manipulation likewise remained the rule. It is Galen who described his treatment and cure of a patrician's hand weakness and numbness through manipulation of the seventh cervical vertebra, and there are ample examples of his techniques which usually retain the principle of traction by assistants whilst the physician's hands, feet, or a wooden plank and pad provide the thrust.

THE ARABIAN EMPIRE

The destruction of the Roman Empire and the ensuing Dark Ages led to the near annihilation of Hippocratic medicine. In Europe little survived except monastic formularies – the scraps of paper copied, amended, and handed down from one generation of monks to the next – whilst the great libraries of recorded knowledge suffered pillage and fire or were simply abandoned. It was the Byzantine empire, able to hold itself together during those turbulent centuries, and the birth of a dynamic force from the Arabian peninsula thirsty for knowledge, which kept the sum of Greek and Roman medical knowledge intact. In 435 AD Nestorius, patriarch of Constantinople, was banished to Petra in Arabia for heresy. Taking with him a great and learned following, his disciples later established not only their creed but a number of schools across Asia Minor, which taught classical Graeco-Roman medicine, including manipulation.

Three centuries later, as the new Arabian civilization carved out its empire from the borders of China to northern Spain, it eagerly adopted Graeco-Roman medicine. In 760–70 AD the Caliph of Baghdad lured many Nestorian physicians to his newly-formed schools of healing; Hunain translated most of the works of Galen into Arabic, and his school translated most of the Hippocratic texts; and such was the Arabian respect for classical learning that, on defeating the Byzantine armies, peace was secured with a camel-train of manuscripts sent from the libraries of Constantinople to Baghdad.

Physicians practised Hippocratic medicine throughout the new Arabian empire. The volumes of Abu 'Ali al-Husain ibn 'Abdullah ibn Sin (Avicenna), and of Abu-l-Qasim (Abulcasius) were translated back into Latin to be used as a standard text in Europe until the seventeenth century. Both include references to manipulation based on the familiar technique of assisted traction and thrust, and one method was modified by Abu-l-Qasim, using a wooden mallet pressed against the spine in place of his hand.

RETURN TO EUROPE

Graeco-Roman medicine returned to Europe through the new tenth century medical faculty at the university of Salerno. Known as the *Collegium Hippocraticum*, it was the first medical school in Europe, and the University's Constantine the African imported countless Arabian manuscripts to which he devoted his life in translation. As they gradually returned into Europe's cultural heritage, the works originally set down by Hippocrates and Galen became the mainstay of Renaissance medicine. The four-teenth century Guy de Chauliac, and later Ambroise Paré – regarded by many as the father of surgery – describe the use of classical manipulation. Paré, who used these methods extensively on sixteenth century French vineyard workers, saw his physician's role as an intermediary unlocking the body's self-recuperative powers, and his words 'I dressed him and God healed him' reveal a humility it behoves all physicians to follow. It was these powers that Palmer was to name 'Innate Intelligence'.

BONESETTERS OF FOLK MEDICINE

Manipulation in its various forms has been practised in folk medicine across the globe from the dawn of human time. Every culture and continent includes forms of massage or joint mobilization performed by families or individuals living within the community. This often took the form of spinal foot trampling and in some societies was accompanied by elaborate ritual. Manipulation was frequently associated with heated baths or massage. In the Middle East it followed a Turkish Bath, and in Scandinavia it sometimes followed a sauna. In the Far East it was used by the barber, when neck manipulation accompanied a haircut. Captain Cook was cured of his sciatica by the massage and lumbar joint 'cracking' of Tahitian women. Manipulation and massage have played an important part in the lives of ordinary folk for centuries, and it is perhaps because of its association with the lower echelons of society that it has been shunned by orthodox medicine. Medicine preferred the more violent and dramatic methods of Hippocrates set down for centuries in the written word, and used them for dealing with the deformities of scoliosis and kyphosis.

The art of Hippocratic manipulation remained virtually unchanged until the time of Palmer himself. His book, *The Science, Art and Philosophy of Chiropractic*, published in 1910, includes an early photograph of the French surgeon Calot manipulating a patient's spine while assistants apply traction. However, more humane methods had been evolving over the centuries within folk medicine, and many a bonesetter found fame and fortune through an ability to cure where established medicine had failed. The French physician Lieutaud, writing on joint problems in 1761, admitted: 'I don't know why the Doctors usually are not very lucky with these cases; they leave them to "les rebouteax" (bonesetters).' Lieutaud adopted some of these techniques for himself, usually with great success.

The first book to be written on the subject in Latin was Friar Morton's *The Compleat Bone-Setter*, and this was 'Revifed, Englifed and Enlarged' by Robert Turner in 1656. Early the next century one of the most colourful but controversial figures was 'Cross-Eyed Sally', Mrs Sarah Mapp of Epsom, to whom English society flocked until her addiction to alcohol drove her to penury. A play was written in her honour entitled *The Husband's Relief, or the Female Bone-Setter and the Worm Doctor*. As if to rub salt into old wounds, a popular song derided her medical opponents:

> *You surgeons of London who puzzle your pates*
> *To ride in your coaches and purchase estates*
> *Give over for shame, for your pride has a fall*
> *The doctress of Epsom has outdone you all.*

Bonesetters entered the periphery of medicine fleetingly in the early nineteenth century through the articles of Edward Harrison in the *London Medical and Physical Journal*. For the twenty years before he moved to London in 1817 Harrison had practised in Lincolnshire, a county famed for its bonesetters. In spite of royal patronage he was opposed by his medical colleagues, and in 1828 successfully defended himself in court against charges brought by the Royal College of Physicians to oust him from London. But he remained ostracized by the medical establishment until his death ten years later.

In spite of the unfavourable attitude bestowed upon Harrison, bonesetting continued to hover at the fringes of orthopaedic medicine. Papers on the subject appeared in medical journals throughout the nineteenth century. In 1882 the British Medical Association even included a discussion at their fiftieth annual meeting. The highly respected surgeon, Sir James Paget, exhorted his colleagues: 'Learn then to imitate what is good and avoid what is bad in the practice of bonesetting. Wise it is to learn from your enemy.' Sir James cannot be faulted in seeking to expand into the realms of physical therapy, but his regard for the manipulative practitioner as an enemy has changed little within official medical quarters during the last hundred years.

The techniques developed by bonesetters, although crude, rarely called for the use of assistants, were quick and usually painless, and often worked where other methods had failed. Before the professions of chiropractic and osteopathy challenged the role of the bonesetter, Sir Herbert Barker brought a measure of respectability to the practice that had till then been sorely lacking. In spite of patronage from the highest levels of British society and a knighthood in 1922 for his services, Sir Herbert bore the same label of charlatan and quack bestowed on his forebears by the medical fraternity. Although his friend Dr Frederick Axham had been struck off the medical register for 'infamous conduct' in acting as his anaesthetist, Barker's gentle persistence eventually paid off. In July 1936, when well into retirement, he demonstrated and lectured to over a hundred surgeons of the British Orthopaedic Association at St Thomas's Hospital in London. Although not considered a respectable form of medicine for another three decades, the simple techniques inspired by Barker and others now entered British orthopaedic medicine, at a time when medical osteopathy, pioneered by Cyriax and others, was gaining the ascendancy.

In the same year that Barker lectured to the British Orthopaedic

Association there were unsuccessful moves to register osteopathy as a new profession in Britain. Osteopathy was in the process of replacing and assimilating bonesetting across the land, but the fledgling chiropractic profession in Britain feared for its very existence. Fiercely preserving their philosophical differences (see Chapter 7), the chiropractors raised the strongest objections. Cyriax and many other British medical osteopaths never forgave them for their stand, so much so that much of their writing still reflects the vehemence of their feelings against the chiropractic profession today.

THE AMERICAN STIMULUS

In America bonesetting arrived from Sweden, Poland, Russia, Germany, Austria, Ireland, and Britain. All these nations had strong bonesetting traditions. As folk medicine it was also firmly entrenched within the indigenous Indian population. The influx of such a diverse range of immigrants gave great scope for the cross-fertilization of techniques and ideas.

One of the earliest books to arise from this melting pot was Waterman Sweet's *An Essay on the Science of Bonesetting*. Written in 1829, it received a mixed reception from the establishment in spite of being widely read. Adopted by those medical physicians who had experienced the successes of the bonesetter, it was still being castigated as quackery by medical opponents thirty years later. Waterman Sweet had descended from a family of bonesetters who had practised in Rhode Island for much of the eighteenth century and well into the nineteenth. Such families were to be found throughout America, which was to become the birthplace of the two major successors to bonesetting, osteopathy and chiropractic.

Chapter 7

A PROFESSION EMERGES

I have never considered it beneath my dignity to do anything to relieve human suffering. *Daniel D. Palmer* (1845–1913), on being jailed in 1906 for practising chiropractic without a medical licence

THE BIRTH OF CHIROPRACTIC

The early years of chiropractic were not without pain as the fledgling profession fought within its own ranks and against osteopathy, and struggled for breath against a medical establishment determined to stifle it at birth. The hostility of Sir James Paget in England towards bonesetting was playful banter compared to the vicious thrashing meted out against chiropractic by American medicine. Here the harsh realities of prison spurred the pioneers of chiropractic to espouse their new cause with an evangelical zeal.

The Palmer family were the first to suffer. In 1903 Palmer's son B.J. was charged with practising medicine without a licence but the case was never concluded. It was Daniel Palmer, father of chiropractic, who became its first martyr. Incarcerated in jail in 1906, aged 61, Palmer became the first of many thousands to suffer fines or imprisonment in the cause of chiropractic.

In 1921 more than 450 Californian chiropractors chose jail rather than a fine, many marching to the court house defiantly singing *Onward Christian Soldiers*. The popular slogan 'Go to jail for chiropractic' was already well established in California, and the Alameda County Chiropractors Association went as far as forbidding their members to pay fines imposed by the courts. Many chiropractors developed a dual practice, serving one group of patients while at liberty and another during their frequent periods of captivity.

Daniel David Palmer was born in a log cabin at Port Perry, eastern Ontario, in 1845. His father was the community shoe-maker and schoolmaster, and was of Anglo-German extraction. His mother was of Scottish and Irish parentage. He passed his first forty years seemingly with little direction, in spite of a contemporary from his schooldays declaring: 'We all thought that Daniel Palmer would do great things.' Another recollected: 'Dan Palmer was a very popular boy, strong, merry and excep-tionally keen-minded. He was always interested in bones and the structure of bodies and used to collect bones of dogs and other animals.'

Daniel David Palmer (1845–1913)

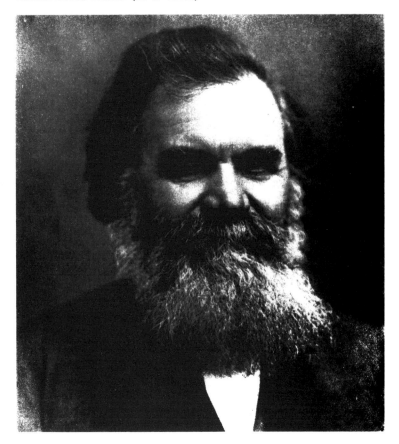

With his younger brother Thomas, and with two dollars between them, the 20-year old Daniel set off on foot to the United States border. Whilst Thomas prospered in his adopted country, Daniel drifted through a variety of occupations. At one time a schoolteacher and at another an itinerant trader, he went through a series of erratic business ventures in his early years which included fruit farming, bee-keeping, and the development and marketing of a heavy-cropping large black raspberry he named 'Sweet Home'. He sold his nursery in 1881 to move to the new town of What Cheer in eastern Iowa, where his son Bartlett Joshua (B.J.) was born, and there he established a grocery specializing in golden carp and other exotic fish. Medical critics later enjoyed laying the foundations of chiropractic at the feet of an 'itinerant grocer', or in another instance a 'fish-peddler', while they chose to pay no heed to his grasp of nineteenth-century medical and scientific knowledge, gleaned from an avid study of the sources then available.

While in What Cheer Palmer first read of the renowned magnetic healer Paul Caster of Ottumwa, Iowa, and at the age of 41 he turned his back on commerce by diving eagerly into the study of anatomy and physiology. Opening a practice in Burlington, Iowa, he drew patients from throughout the American Midwest, and later moved to Brady Street, Davenport.

Chiropractic traces its birth to 18 September 1895, when Harvey Lillard, the janitor of the Ryan building in which Palmer practised, received the first chiropractic 'adjustment'. Lillard reported that 'when he was exerting himself in a cramped, stooping position, he felt something give way in his back and immediately became deaf.' Palmer surmised that if his patient's deafness 17 years before had been linked to this spinal accident, which he located at the fourth thoracic vertebra, then he could restore Lillard's hearing by reversing that process. He set about this task and 'racked it into position by using the spinous process as a lever and soon the man could hear as before'. Underlining the logic and predetermination of this manoeuvre, Palmer emphasized: 'It was accomplished with an object in view, and the result expected was obtained. There was nothing crude about this adjustment; it was specific.'

With the curing of Harvey Lillard's deafness a new branch of medicine was born. In one lifetime chiropractic was to sweep not only through North America but throughout the rest of the Western world.

MEDICINE IN PALMER'S AMERICA

To understand why Palmer's new brand of medicine was able to germinate and later thrive we must look at the provision of health care in the nineteenth century in his native land. The picture we have been given by Hollywood film producers of the itinerant peddlers selling their alcoholic elixirs from covered wagons is not far from the truth.

In many states there were no laws to lay down who could or could not practise medicine and in some areas physicians were barely literate. Often amounting to a full attack on the bodily system, medicine's liking for blood-letting, purges, and massive doses of calomel drew an understandable public reaction, and surgeons were frequently feared and suspected. The story of Kentucky surgeon Ephraim McDowell, who performed the first successful removal of an ovarian cyst, reflects nineteenth-century popular mistrust for medicine. In 1809, in the most primitive conditions, he operated on the valiant Mrs Crawford while she sang hymns and the town's lynch mob clamoured outside for his blood.

Before the American Civil War, Ladies Physiological Societies had sprung up to impart a knowledge of basic human biology to their members, whose distrust of conventional medicine had brought them together. Fanny Wright's People's Hall of Science in New York offered enlightenment courses in physiology to overcome the ordinary person's ignorance of those bodily functions that medicine preferred to conceal. The movement to democratize medicine was further boosted by Samuel Thomson's Friendly Botanical Societies, which spread herbal remedies throughout the United States. It was so successful that those states with medical licensing laws either repealed or relaxed them in the 1830s and 1840s. Eclectic colleges and hospitals sprang up to rival the allopathic establishment, aided in this by the homoeopaths, who were larger and better organized, with their strong European traditions.

Meanwhile the seeds were already being sown for the destruction of this popular movement when the American dentist Wells used nitric oxide ('laughing gas') for an extraction in the year Palmer was born. This was followed rapidly by ether and then chloroform, silencing the terrified screams of the operating theatre and allowing both time and precision to enter the realms of surgery. When an appreciation of asepsis followed, the process was complete, although – as with many innovations – valuable time was lost by the narrow-minded attitude of established medicine. In 1847 the Austrian doctor Semmelweis's insistence upon hygiene at childbirth was cruelly ridiculed, so much so that it led to his depressive illness and untimely death. Lister's use of carbolic acid and phenol sprays twenty years later, although equally derided, made survival from surgery the norm, rather than the exception it had been till then.

Pasteur's germ theory and Virchow's work on the cell led to conventional medicine regarding disease as a series of pathogens invading the body in military fashion. The body became the battle-ground and the enemy was met with more and more complex drugs designed specifically to disarm or kill off the foe. When the battle was being lost surgery was often chosen, and the battle-ground itself cut away to isolate and destroy the invasive force.

Conventional medicine allied itself closely to scientific discovery and patronage. Advances in public health, drainage and uncontaminated fresh water supplies, clean childbirth, and an understanding of how the major diseases were transmitted were allied to the best dietary and hygiene concepts of the popular eclectic movement. It ceased to be common for women to die in labour, and diseases like cholera and typhoid, denied entry to the water supplies, came under control. Mistrust and fear, which had earlier embodied the public perception of conventional medicine, were replaced by total faith and adulation as science became the new god of the twentieth century, casting out concepts of spirituality and the frailty of humankind.

As this newborn faith in humankind's potential for self determination took control, and allopathic medicine donned its new mask of humanity, so the eclectic and homoeopathic schools and hospitals waned. In America the forerunner of today's conventional medicine absorbed from its opponents their concepts of diet and hygiene, so that as the twentieth century approached allopathic medicine appeared to offer the greatest hope, while eclectic and homoeopathic medicine now appeared outmoded and irrelevant.

Laws to define medicine and to regulate its practice sprang up throughout America, limiting healthcare to allopathy in most states. Provision was made for the inclusion of all practising physicians of whatever background and persuasion, usually with the proviso that they should have been in practice for the preceding five years. Iowa closed its doors in 1886, five years too early to embrace Palmer within the medical establishment he would later defy. Had he been eligible it is still unlikely that Palmer, with his wilful determination to defy conformity, would have seized the chance to register as a medical physician – unlike other magnetic healers. It was this determination to ignore the establishment that put him beyond the pale, and when he openly challenged allopathy with his chiropractic philosophy his new-found system was met with opposition which had all the subtlety of a sledgehammer cracking a walnut.

THE CHRISTENING OF CHIROPRACTIC

Seeking a name for his discovery Palmer turned to his friend, patient, and student, the Rev. Samuel H. Weed to provide a suitable classical title. Weed chose the words *cheiri* ('a hand') and *praktikos* ('performed') to derive *chiropractic*. Explaining this title, Palmer was to write: 'CHIROPRACTIC (ki-ro-prak-tic) is from two Greek words . . . done by hand – a hand practitioner – One who repairs – One who adjusts.'

DIFFERENCES FROM OSTEOPATHY

As an avid reader there can be little doubt that Palmer was aware of the work of Andrew Taylor Still, who had established his first osteopathic school in the neighbouring state of Missouri in 1892. In later years Palmer wrote: 'Chiropractic resembles osteopathy more so than any other method; yet they are different as day is from night,' adding: 'The philosophies of Osteopathy and Chiropractic are radically and entirely different.' Of these philosophies he stated: 'Osteopathy is founded upon the circulation of the blood, whereas, Chiropractic is founded upon the quality of nerve tissues and its ability to transmit functioning impulses.' Describing his chiropractic methods Palmer declared them to be: 'unique, unlike any used by any other school; they are direct as desired by a chiropractor who should make a specific move for a specific purpose with an aim in view'.

THE BIRTH OF OSTEOPATHY

Still developed his system of medicine after the all too familiar story of allopathic disaster, when three of his own children were lost to meningitis. Following a vision in 1874 he 'flung to the breeze the banner of osteopathy'. Although he had attended some lessons at the Kansas City College of Physicians and Surgeons he appears on no graduate list and took no final examinations, but unlike Palmer he registered as a member of the medical profession. He was therefore able to propagate osteopathy from within the safe confines of a registered medical profession, unlike Palmer who lacked this apparent advantage and became the first chiropractic martyr to medicine. Yet when Palmer died in 1913 it was in the knowledge that the profession he had founded was growing from strength to strength. When Still died a few years later he had watched his profession expand with initial promise only to be thwarted by ridicule and partial absorption by the medical fraternity within whose confines he lay.

In England, Still's osteopathy was preserved by the foresight of Martin Littlejohn, whose British School of Osteopathy, established in 1917, ensured a strong and independent foothold in British society. In America osteopathy was largely assimilated by medicine; during the 1930s the American Medical Association (AMA) granted recognition to six osteopathic colleges, basing this status on regular inspection. By the 1960s the typical American osteopath had turned his back on manipulation, preferring the prescription or injection of drugs, and enjoying the full title, privileges, and status of a Doctor of Medicine. Although the traditional American osteopaths are belatedly fighting back, theirs is an uphill struggle.

When the AMA's House of Delegates resolved that each state medical society was free to accept osteopaths as professional equals in 1961, the way was paved for one of the most influential osteopathic colleges to disavow its parentage. That year the California College of Osteopathic Physicians and Surgeons decided by a majority vote of one to name itself the University of California College of Medicine, Irvine, and all osteopathy degrees were retrospectively converted to M.D. degrees upon return of a Doctor of Osteopathy (D.O.) certificate and a small fee. This was accompanied by the merging of the California State Medical and Osteopathic Societies, and from that time a block was placed upon the granting of any future osteopathic licences in the state of California. This action completed the process described by Morris Fishbein in 1925 when, as editor of the *Journal of the American Medical Association*, he wrote: 'Osteopathy is essentially a method of entering medicine by the back door.' Chiropractic could not match even this begrudging acceptance, for Fishbein continued: 'Chiropractic by contrast is an attempt to arrive through the cellar.'

Whilst the attitude of medicine towards osteopathy had initially been hostile, its opposition to chiropractic was openly vehement. *Agents provocateurs* were recruited by local medical societies to become the patients of chiropractors, and would then testify to the courts that the chiropractor had made a medical diagnosis or delivered a treatment. One might have expected in these circumstances the strengthening of ties between the two forms of manipulative medicine as they faced their giant allopathic foe, yet this was not to be.

The osteopaths bitterly complained that Palmer had not only stolen Still's philosophical and metaphysical concepts, but his phraseology as well. Chiropractors have hotly denied this, but whatever the truth both claimed to have discovered a complete system of medicine. They referred to their respective seats of learning as the 'Fountainhead', and coined the maxim taught to every student of chiropractic and osteopathy: 'Find it, fix it, leave it alone.' Still's Law of the Artery, that diseases follow from a reduction of blood flow, was matched by Palmer's Law of the Nerve, that reduced nerve flow and not blood circulation leads to disease. In spite of reports of secret meetings between the two founders at Clinton, Iowa, reconciliation was not to be, and osteopathy's attempts to distance itself from chiropractic led to closer and closer flirtations with the medical establishment.

CHIROPRACTIC DIVISION

If early chiropractors were unable to get along with osteopaths they were equally unable to get along with themselves. Persecuted by medical ridicule and legal prosecution, the pioneer chiropractor needed an unshakeable faith, a very thick skin, and a stubborn heart – qualities which rarely combine with diplomacy and tact. When Daniel Palmer was incarcerated in jail he left his 25-year-old son Bartlett Joshua in command of his

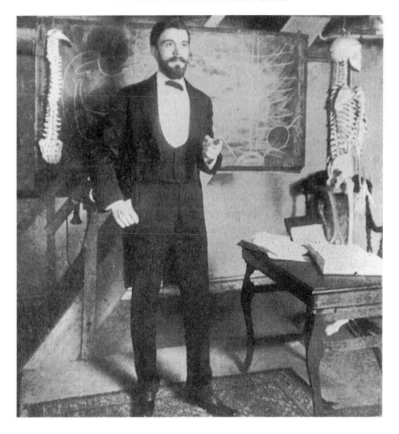

B.J. Palmer lecturing at the Palmer School of Chiropractic, 1906. His dynamism ensured the survival of chiropractic

ailing Palmer Infirmary and Chiropractic Institute and its twelve students. B.J. took out a personal loan to pay off its $US8,000 debts and soon turned it into a profitable concern. Later that year he purchased it from his father for the sum of $US2196.79 and incorporated it as the Palmer School of Chiropractic.

From this position B.J. was to dominate the chiropractic profession until his death in 1961. An imaginative, determined and independent thinker like his father, he added to these qualities remarkable organizational, commercial, and leadership skills, terming himself the 'Developer' of chiropractic where his father was the 'Discoverer'. Often at loggerheads, the two rarely communicated, and – possibly as a result of striking his head on the concrete floor of his cell – Daniel became increasingly difficult to live with.

Daniel left Davenport at the end of 1906 and spent the next seven years establishing schools, usually disastrously, as he travelled through the Indian Territories, California, Oregon, and eventually Canada, before spending the last few weeks of his life in Los Angeles. A grand public reunion designed to reconcile the followings of father and son went severely awry on 20 August 1913, when Daniel stormed off claiming he had been run down by a car driven by his son. No opportunity was lost by dissenting camps when, after Daniel's death in 1913, a charge of murder was brought against B.J. together with a $US32,000 claim for damages. Brought to trial 14 months later, the court heard that the accident had probably never happened, and as Daniel had died of typhoid and not from the effects of physical injury, the judge dismissed the case, leaving B.J. a free man.

EARLY EDUCATION

Before his death Daniel Palmer had seen dozens of chiropractic schools sprout up across the United States, and although some were undoubtedly little more than diploma mills others were of a high standard for their day. Indeed, there was nothing extraordinary in this diversity, as Abraham Flexner's 1910 investigation into medical education for the Carnegie Foundation had revealed. Writing later, Flexner described how:

> Loose and shifting bands of practising physicians, calling themselves a faculty, tried to impart, chiefly by lectures, to heterogenous uneducated groups of students the empirical knowledge – sound and unsound – which they themselves possessed. First and last, American towns have produced over four hundred such medical schools. The teaching of medicine on these terms was, directly in cash, and indirectly in prestige, a profitable business.

In the early 1920s conventional medicine virtually eradicated such institutions, and economic reality forced the hand of chiropractic shortly after. As the weaker colleges merged with the stronger in the mid 1920s, a uniform pattern of chiropractic education was beginning to emerge.

CHIROPRACTIC AND X-RAYS

Within three years of taking over the directorship of the Palmer School, B.J. introduced one key element that was to identify chiropractic from other forms of manipulative medicine. In the year that chiropractic was born Roentgen discovered how to generate X-rays with a cathode tube, leading the way for

B.J. Palmer examining X-rays. His introduction of radiographic analysis in 1909 was a catalyst for the development of many new specific chiropractic techniques

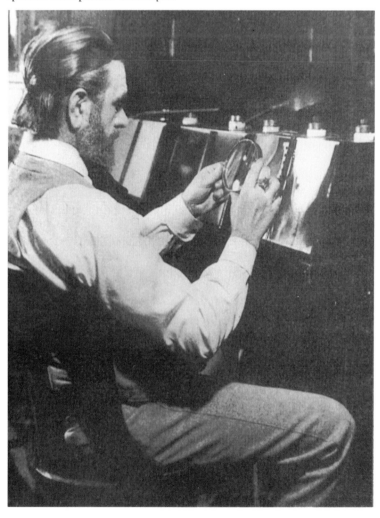

radiographic diagnosis to develop. Acquiring a unit in 1909, B.J. established a laboratory the following year. His enthusiasm for X-ray analysis prompted a rapid development of techniques, and a number of standard radiographic positions for the study of bony structures were pioneered by chiropractors in those early years.

Not only were chiropractors now equipped to identify destructive bone diseases and bone thinning (osteoporosis), but they could appreciate the multiple variables of structure that provide the asymmetries which differentiate each one of us from our neighbour. The next step was the development of even more specific manipulative techniques – which chiropractors call 'adjustment' – to suit every need. These range from gentle non-force approaches to the light high-speed 'toggle recoil', using the individual shapes of joint surfaces revealed on X-ray to determine the most effective adjustment. Although D.D. Palmer had called for chiropractic adjustment to be specific, the profession was now able to develop a myriad of highly specialized techniques as a result of radiography, and the consequent attention to detail at a specific vertebral level.

STRAIGHTS AND MIXERS

Like his father, B.J. Palmer's attention to vertebral detail and the development of specific adjusting techniques led him to brand as heretical any approach which was not concentrated on the chiropractic adjustment alone. On this subject Daniel had written:

> A chiropractor who comprehends the Principles of this Science will have no use for adjuncts. Just in proportion as he lacks knowledge and confidence (the two go together) he will use remedies, become a mixer. The more he mixes the less use he has for chiropractic.

However, there were many who disagreed. They argued that other methods of natural healing could be successfully used alongside chiropractic to enhance the power of the adjustment, and they introduced physical therapy, diet, colonic irrigation, specific exercises, and the like, to their practice. These practitioners both Palmers condemned as 'Mixers', calling their band of faithful purists the 'Straights'. Rivalries persist today in the United States with the Federation of Straight Chiropractic Organizations forming a tiny minority, whilst the two giant organizations, the American Chiropractic Association (ACA) and the International Chiropractic Association (ICA) allow their members to use adjunctive therapies.

Controversy within chiropractic dates back to the rivalries between the three great pioneers of the profession, a group one chiropractic historian reverently termed the 'Trinity of Giants'. D.D. Palmer the 'Discoverer' argued that disease was an alteration in the tone of the nervous system brought about by 'impingement', or stretching, at the point where the nerve leaves the spinal column. His son B.J. the 'Developer' claimed the cause to be direct pressure on the nerve and dispensed 'Pure Straight and Unadulterated' chiropractic from his school, which he hailed as 'universally recognized as the hub of all things chiropractic'. Willard Carver, a lawyer from the Indian Territories and one time legal adviser to Daniel, was the other early combatant. Calling himself the 'Constructor' he was often at loggerheads with both Palmers, and established several successful schools teaching his 'Scientific Catechism'. Many other dynamic characters entered the scene in these formative years.

A dispute with B.J. in 1906 provoked the medically qualified Arthur Forster to form his own National School. Forster later criticized B.J. for claiming that 'all disease is due to subluxations of the vertebrae and that all diseases could be eradicated by adjustment of the vertebrae'. Forster's powerful influence and success helped keep in balance some of the more extravagant claims of the Palmer School. Another medical chiropractor, Alvah Gregory, who had teamed up with Daniel to form a school in Oklahoma City shortly after Palmer's release from jail, was to argue that the vertebral subluxation was not a displacement but a 'relaxation of spinal ligaments'. This disagreement drove both apart, yet modern understanding identifies ligamentous instability as being one of the more frequent causes of spinal problems.

STRUGGLE FOR SURVIVAL

In spite of the many schools springing up across the United States in chiropractic's first three decades, B.J. Palmer remained its greatest influence, guiding its development through its most critical times. Without his dynamic organizational capacities, his massive personal investment – given without financial gain – his charismatic nature, and the reputation of his Palmer School, this disparate and squabbling band of early chiropractors would have been effectively annihilated by the end of the Great Depression. Palmer's school boasted some 3,100 students in 1922, each regarding him with the reverence and awe reserved for a cult figure. In his white linen suit and sporting a long, black silk bowtie hung halfway to his chest, this magical figure with shoulder length flowing hair knew how to capture and hold his student audience.

Preaching Pure Chiropractic and castigating Mixers, Palmer saw himself as providing through chiropractic a panacea to cure all the world's ills. He exhorted students at his Davenport Fountainhead to 'Get The Big Idea' and sent them out not only across the Americas but to all corners of the globe with a youthful burning zeal. Brought before the courts for practising medicine, many would claim that they were neither making a diagnosis nor treating disease. Their adjustments were 're-aligning' the spine so that 'Innate Intelligence' – nature's life force – could flow through the nerves and bring about full health. They based their beliefs on B.J.'s simple Garden Hose theory; as a kink in the hose will cut down the flow of water, so a vertebral displacement will press on the nerve and reduce nerve flow.

Such simplistic ideas exemplified Palmer's attempt to distance chiropractic from any possible confusion with medicine at a time when many of the American state laws were highly prohibitive of non-allopathic medicine. He argued that he was not diagnosing or treating disease, but encouraging health. Like encouraging good diet, adjustment was a means to full health and not the administration of medicine. It was these fervent zealots who were keeping chiropractic alive through the Great Depression when, in 1929, only 300 students were enrolled at Palmer School and its financial affairs were under the control of the First National Bank of Davenport.

In those states where chiropractic was most under attack from medical licensing laws thousands of chiropractors were indicted. Medical writer Arthur Geiger noted in 1942 that there had been 15,000 prosecutions in the first thirty years of chiropractic's existence. One-fifth had resulted in conviction. Records kept by the Universal Chiropractic Association show that by 1927 the Association had acted in the defence of their members in 3,300 court actions. For most of the 1920s and 1930s the *Chiropractor and Clinical Journal* carried lists of its 'crusaders' who were behind bars, exhorting their readers to correspond with them to keep their spirits up. It was their burning belief in the rightness of the cause that kept the embers of chiropractic aglow in the economic hardships before and after the Second World War, and which allowed it to burst into flame again in the recovery years of the 1950s and 1960s. In those two decades the early philosophies were successfully blended with modern scientific knowledge to produce the quality chiropractic we know today.

EARLY RESEARCH

It would be wrong to leave the impression that B.J. totally rejected science. He was fascinated by new gadgetry, and we have seen his part in the introduction of X-ray diagnosis. He was also responsible for devising the neurocalometer (NCM) to record the minute temperature differences which accompany a subluxation (joint malfunction). These differences can largely be detected by the skilled examining hand, but the neurocalometer needle dramatically demonstrated them visually on a dial, and later versions graphically recorded them on a paper roll as the instrument was drawn down the spine from the skull to the base of the vertebral column. B.J.'s commitment to his new instrument was total, as he claimed that: 'No chiropractor can practise chiropractic without an NCM . . . no chiropractor can render an efficient, competent or honest service without the NCM.' Its introduction, at his 1924 homecoming lecture entitled 'The Hour has Struck', split the profession. It lost him many of his old purist supporters who claimed that because the instrument was not analysis 'done by hand' it could not be considered chiropractic. Worse than that old argument was the accusation that it was an extortionate attempt to ransom the profession. The cost of leasing the instrument from the Palmer School was a $US2,500 licence (later reduced to $US150) plus a monthly rental of $US5, and Palmer threatened that if insufficient numbers were taken up he would hand it over to the barbers who would then replace chiropractors. In spite of his preposterously histrionic behaviour at the 1924 homecoming, it is estimated that a thousand were leased during those days, with another thousand being dispersed in the coming year. It remained a popular tool for forty years, although few use it today.

Less practical was B.J.'s Electroencephaloneuromentimpo-graph. Modified from Hans Berger's electroencephalograph, it was housed in a two-ton steel box, 28 feet long, 14 feet wide, and 8 feet high (8.5×4.3×2.5m). The whole structure was elaborately shielded externally with reinforced concrete walling and earthed internally with copper mosquito net wiring in an attempt to eradicate electrical variables in the environment. The instrument measured the conduction of brainwaves through the central nervous system, and with it Palmer hoped to identify and measure the mental impulse flow which lay at the core of his philosophy.

The museum of osteological specimens at Davenport started by Daniel was extensively expanded by B.J. to include what the American Medical Association's Council on Medical Education and Hospitals called 'without doubt the best collection of human spines in existence'. He X-rayed his collection of Egyptian mummies to demonstrate the osseous diseases which plagued this ancient aristocracy.

B.J. established a clinical research centre in 1935 with the most up-to-date diagnostic equipment available. Into this he received the most difficult medical cases, in an endeavour to show that chiropractic could win where allopathic medicine had already given up hope. He initiated research into the effects of adjust-ment on blood pressure, heart rate, respiration and other bodily functions, and published hundreds of papers demonstrating the superiority of chiropractic adjustment to the medical approach. Much of his work would not withstand modern scientific scrutiny, but it should be remembered that at the time medical science had yet to perform its first clinical trial. On a few occasions his enthusiasm for the cause led him towards a bias and selectivity which sadly brings into question the validity of the rest of his work, yet the seeds of research planted by him sixty years ago were reaped in the 1970s and 1980s when a small band of researchers applied scientific principles to the examination of chiropractic theories, this time to dramatic and positive effect.

DECLINE OF PALMER'S INFLUENCE

When choosing 'The Hour has Struck' as the title for his 1924 address B. J. Palmer believed he was ushering in a new era for chiropractic. Yet it was not to be the hour of the neurocalometer but the eleventh hour of his own waning influence that he heralded. He left the cream of his Palmer College faculty disenchanted, so much so that within two years many had left to form Lincoln College in Indianapolis. Only a few chiropractic colleges were to survive the 1930s and 1940s. These were by and large the soundest colleges, not only financially but in the quality of their instruction. By his own hand Palmer had lost effective control of a chiropractic movement which had outgrown the need for single personalities.

Shortly before the Second World War, B.J.'s insistence that subluxations of the top two vertebrae were the key to full health led to another major revolt. This technique, termed the Hole-In-One or Palmer Specific, and later the Upper Cervical Specific, relied on careful X-ray measurement and correctly applied toggle recoil adjustment to either the atlas or axis. B.J. now felt the need to challenge the very roots of chiropractic. Whereas his father, describing the first chiropractic adjustment on Harvey Lillard, had asserted quite clearly: 'I replaced the displaced fourth dorsal vertebra by one move, which restored his hearing fully,' B.J. was now to reiterate time and time again: 'It was not the fourth dorsal vertebra but the axis which was adjusted in Harvey Lillard.'

Although B.J. Palmer remained the most awe-inspiring figure in the chiropractic movement until his death, he could not prevent its inevitable drift away from the rigid strait-jacket he had placed upon it in harder times. Dr H.M. Hines, Director of Technique at Palmer School, laid down a revised policy for his department in 1956. The following year it received B.J.'s signature and came into force in 1958. The new programme directed students to: 'Compare the merits of upper cervical specific technique and lower spine adjusting . . . This will lead eventually to integration of the entire spinal column on a specific rather than a general adjusting basis.'

The *Journal of the Canadian Chiropractic Association* commented:

> This would seem to be a most important step toward unity within our profession. Everyone knows that differences over techniques have been one of the greatest stumbling blocks to chiropractic professional progress. By incorporating full spine adjusting into 'the new technic curriculum for PSC', the Palmer School has taken a great step forward toward solving our technic difficulties.

The school was now ready to begin teaching adjustment of the 'full spine', as espoused by Daniel David Palmer and as taught at the other major chiropractic colleges, which between them now graduated the lion's share of the new chiropractic profession.

B.J. PALMER'S CONTRIBUTION

When B.J.'s son David took on the Palmer mantle the period of mourning was brief. It was no longer a time to look back at the past but a time to grow into a new era. In his lifetime B.J.'s vigorous defence of his beloved profession against the overt attacks of allopathic medicine had projected him as the natural leader of the profession. His personal appearance in law courts across the length and breadth of the United States of America swayed many a jury. Chiropractic, he argued, could not be conceived as medicine, which attacked disease with external agents. Unlike medicine it had no need for medical diagnosis. Detection and adjustment of the spinal subluxation provided humankind with the most powerful means of resisting disease known, building up nature's own defences from within so that disease had no foothold to gain.

B.J.'s boundless energy in lobbying key national figures, many of whom were personal friends, gave to chiropractic allies that helped to secure and protect it at the highest levels of American society during its bleakest hours. At his home he hosted Presidents Calvin Coolidge, Herbert Hoover, and Harry S. Truman, and future President Ronald Reagan worked as a broadcaster on his WOC radio station during his early career.

B.J.'s foresight in establishing only the second commercial station in the United States gave him time to develop and perfect the skills of media selling. His ability to package and market chiropractic gave it a truly powerful public image, and ensured that, in the eyes of the average American citizen, B.J. Palmer was the embodiment of chiropractic. Although his personal intervention often created division and controversy within the profession, there can be little doubt that by imprinting chiropractic upon the social awareness of Americans, this amazing man achieved more for the chiropractic profession than any other individual in its history.

A MATURING PROFESSION

The period after the Second World War was one of regrowth and consolidation as educational standards were established and chiropractic tenets put to closer scientific scrutiny. Training now demanded four years of full-time education and the call of D.D. Palmer to study conscientiously and to examine chiropractic scientifically was taken to heart.

More and more states made provision for chiropractic licensure, yet the public continued to be outraged by examples of American justice meted out to chiropractors in backward states. In 1949 husband and wife Mack and Kitty Scallon served time in separate maximum security prisons in spite of support from the Kennedy family. Kitty wrote to a friend on hearing of the death of B.J.'s wife, who had steered the chiropractic course beside him:

> I felt down-hearted when the news came that Mabel died, but I would always perk up when I thought of chiropractic and the many people it had helped . . . and then I'd throw my shoulders back and be ready and willing to make any sacrifice to help free our beloved science.

Prosecutions continued throughout the 1950s and early 1960s, mainly in New York and Massachusetts, but soon these states fell to the march of progress. During 1965 almost half of Louisiana's chiropractors were found guilty of illegally practising medicine. This prompted an energetic defence, culminating in success when the United States Court of Appeals, Fifth Circuit, over-turned the verdict. When licensure was granted by Louisiana in 1974 the legislative process was complete in the USA.

Although now enshrined in law, chiropractic nevertheless needed to regularize its educational base as well. The establishment of the Council on Chiropractic Education which set out to establish minimum standards in the teaching of the medical foundation studies known as basic sciences was achieved in 1947. Full accreditation was granted by the United States government in 1974, setting the highest standards of chiropractic education whilst permitting a leeway in underlying philosophy. What the Council had achieved was a common base-line from which to lay down minimum standards of train-ing in chiropractic and diagnostic studies, and this American standard became the model for chiropractic education worldwide by the end of the 1970s.

Official civil positions reserved in the past for medical graduates have in many states been opened to chiropractors, and some chiropractors are also coroners. At one time both the Senate and House Public Health Committees in the state of Washington were chaired by chiropractors, and chiropractors have become members of a number of statewide Health Co-Ordinating Councils. In 1980 twelve chiropractors were appointed to regional committees of the California Board of Medical Quality Assurance by the State Governor. Chiropractic treatment is now available to patients eligible for state assisted Medicaid and Medicare, and in 1974 Congress earmarked $US2 million for chiropractic research.

In research some of the most convincing results have come from analysis of records held by Workers Compensation Boards. On the advice of their actuaries, who have no axe to grind and whose job is to save money, many private insurance companies have also chosen to include chiropractic care. The process started by Mutual of Omaha in 1951 gradually spread beyond the private sector. In 1974 the Wisconsin Workers Compensation Board completed a study identifying chiropractic as the most economic form of treatment for back pain, and this was repeated in other states. The Californian Workers Compensation Board studied 1,000 cases to learn that, whereas it took medical doctors an average of 32 days to return a man to work, it took chiropractors a mere 15.6 days for comparable injuries. The Oregon Workers Compensation Board found that twice as many of their injured workers were returned to work within a week by chiropractic than by medicine. The most meticulous study, involving all 102,487 Workers' Compensation claims for back-related injuries during Florida's 1985–6 fiscal year, has proved one of the most favourable. It showed that chiropractic patients were less likely to be absent from work for more than seven days. Of those incapacitated for more than a week, 23.2 per cent went on to be hospitalized, whereas 57.7 per cent of medical and 49.3 per cent of osteopathic cases were to receive hospital care. In comparing the total expense of all treatment, medical costs were 83.8 per cent higher than chiropractic in the non-surgery group, and 95.3 per cent higher in the group which included surgery patients. This study, which was published in 1988, has confirmed yet again that chiropractic minimizes prolonged absence from work-related back injuries, and is considerably cheaper.

One of the latest studies to be published in the medical press confirms these findings. Reported in the March 1989 *Western Journal of Medicine*, it was based on a follow-up questionnaire conducted at the Group Health Co-Operative of Puget Sound, a Health Maintenance Organization in the state of Washington. It was found that 48 per cent of low-back pain patients treated by their family medical physician remained unable to resume their normal activities within a week, whereas only 17 per cent of chiropractic patients remained restricted. The total of disability days averaged at 39.7 days for medical patients, and this compared with only 10.8 days for the patients of chiropractors. The report concluded:

> The most profound difference between chiropractors and family physicians is their training and consequent beliefs, attitudes, and behaviours concerning the management of low back pain . . . The results of this study suggest that patients may be more satisfied with the confident and definite approach of chiropractors.

MEDICAL RESTRAINT OF TRADE

In spite of the arrival of chiropractic at the gates of the establishment, it is still subject to skirmishes with the allopathic political machine. A case brought by five Chicago chiropractors headed by Chester Wilk in 1976 against the American Medical Association, nine medical organizations, one hospital association, one hospital accreditation body, and four individuals, for violation of antitrust legislation and restraint of trade has only just been successfully concluded after 11 years. It revealed an organized conspiracy first to contain and then to eliminate chiropractic. Grudgingly medical associations and hospitals conceded by permitting close co-operation with chiropractors, but the AMA, in spite of being forced to publish an admission of guilt, is still fighting on appeal to the bitter end to buy itself time – time in which to train its doctors and physical therapists in the Art and Science of Manipulation so that, in the words of Raymond Chaipin M.D. in the August 1985 edition of *Medical Economics*, 'M.D.s should learn to do manipulation so that money chiropractors are taking can rightfully go into physician's pockets'.

Chapter 8

DEVELOPMENT OF PRINCIPLES AND THEORIES

No man of science could subscribe without qualification to all of Galileo's beliefs, or to all of Newton's beliefs, or to all of his own beliefs of ten years ago. *Lord William Beveridge* (1879–1963)

We have seen how manipulation grew from ancient Greek practice through 2,000 years of stagnation in Europe to be blended with the traditions and art of the bonesetters as chiropractic. Early chiropractic theories may seem backward and simplistic to those with a deep knowledge of neurophysiology, but it must be remembered that in 1895 the science of neurophysiology had barely begun.

THE HUMORAL THEORY OF MEDICINE

The ancient Greek concept of the four humours struggled on with modifications into D. D. Palmer's century, with Robitansky's *Pathological Anatomy* being published three years after Palmer's birth as its curtain-call. Deriving the original doctrine from Empedocles (*circa* 500–430 BC), Aristotle had held that the four primary qualities of matter – heat and cold, dryness and wetness – combined in balanced pairs to form the four elements of air and earth, water and fire. To this concept the Hippocratic Corpus added the theory that mental and physical health was dependent upon the four humours – blood and phlegm, and yellow and black bile – with which they corresponded and were balanced as opposing pairs. The surplus or deficiency of any humour led to illness and was met with measures to depress or stimulate the imbalance.

In about 290 BC Herophilus of Alexandria was the first to recognize the brain as the central organ of the nervous system and the source of intelligence, opposing those philosophers before him who saw the heart as the centre. Some nerves he associated with movement and others with sensation. His contemporary Erasistratus regarded man's higher intelligence as being the property of the brain's convolutions, and saw the contraction of muscles as their response to a 'subtle vapour', or breath, which he termed 'pneuma'.

PNEUMATIC THEORY

Galen accepted the pneumatic theory and elaborated it further. Drawn in during the act of breathing, pneuma followed several processes before being differentiated into 'Natural Spirit' controlling growth and nutrition, the higher grade 'Vital Spirit' charged with the principle of life, and the noblest of all, the 'Animal Spirit' bearing the breath of the soul. Animal spirit was stored in the brain and was carried through the body in hollow nerves to initiate higher functions such as sensation and movement.

The two doctrines of humours and pneuma remained virtually unchallenged until the sixteenth century when Paracelsus first poured scorn on them, but they were to survive in spite of him. Two hundred years were to pass before Stahl (1660–1734) opposed the pneumatic doctrine with his concept that 'Anima', a living force, lay within the body, stimulating the muscles to contract, the glands to secrete, and performing every aspect of internal function, so that when this spiritual force was depleted disease followed. This Vitalist principle was advanced by Robert Whytt's theory that anima guided our intelligence and worked through the brain and nerves.

NERVE FORCE THEORIES

With the work of Galvani (1737–1798), more was learned about electricity during the eighteenth century. William Cullen

(1710–1790) viewed the vital force as being similar to this new-found phenomenon. Calling it *vis medicatrix naturae*, he held that as nerve energy it was responsible for all vital functions, and any disturbance to its flow led to disease. Publishing his *First Lines in the Practice of Physic* in 1776, he claimed that relaxation as well as activity was brought about by the positive involvement of nerve energy, thereby anticipating the autonomic nervous system. His pupil John Brown conceived an opposing view which met with much popularity, but it was not long before people were claiming Brown's theories had 'killed more than the French Revolution'. Cullen, who was a founding father of the Glasgow Medical School, was greatly respected in the medical community and it was his concepts which won through. They led to intense interest being directed to the nervous system and spine as the area in which the origin of disease lay.

Interest in the spine was further generated by Sir Charles Bell's dramatic differentiation of sensory from motor nerves in 1811, and his work was refined by François Magendie in 1822 when he plotted these pathways as they left the spinal cord. Marshall-Hall's work in 1833 introduced the concept of a nerve reflex, and the dramatic discoveries of these great men led to spinal cord pathology being heralded as the obvious cause of most diseases during Palmer's century.

SPINAL IRRITATION

A new term 'Spinal Irritation' was coined by Dr Thomas Brown of Glasgow in 1828 to describe those conditions which were accompanied by pressure tenderness over the spine. Dr Corrigan of Dublin in the *Lancet* called it 'the greatest improvement in practical medicine' in his living memory and added, 'other improvements may have been more brilliant, but there has been none so useful'.

The concept reached America through Dr Isaac Parrish of Philadelphia in 1832, and four years later he was listing the manifestations of spinal irritation in an *American Journal of Medical Sciences* article entitled 'Remarks upon many symptomatic affections which are encountered in cases of irritation of a greater or lesser portion of the spinal marrow'. These included a wide range of common disorders from asthma and diabetes to vertigo, shortness of breath, coughs, colic, and menstrual cramps. The diagnosis was confirmed when spinal tenderness could be linked to a spinal nerve or sympathetic ganglion passing from that vertebral level to the diseased area.

Treatment of spinal irritation bore many similarities to traditional methods in that blistering, leeches, and cauterization were used. However, in this instance, instead of being applied to alter the balance of Humours it was administered as a counter-irritant over the relevant vertebra to encourage flow of Cullen's *vis medicatrix naturae.*

It was galvanism that had triggered Cullen to conceive the nerve force as electrical energy, and a century later it was galvanism that provided a novel means for correcting spinal irritation. In his 1871 *A Treatise on Disease of the Nervous System*, the neurologist William Hammond attributed it to anaemia of the posterior columns of the spinal cord and suggested it should be remedied by a galvanic current passed across the offending vertebra. It is quite possible that this contemporary thinking led to osteopathy's founder, Andrew Taylor Still, laying down his Rule of the Artery. He held that disruption to the blood supply of the spinal cord or other tissues led to malfunction and disease – a claim that was countered by Daniel David Palmer's Rule of the Nerve.

It is possible that Palmer was influenced by the ideas of Dr Edward Harrison, published in the 1820s amidst much medical scepticism. He introduced the idea that vertebrae could over-stretch, allowing them to move too much. This induced pressure or stretching of spinal nerves 'by which their energies are impaired, interrupted, or morbidly affected'. He went on to explain: 'A very slight or partial pressure on the nerve or nerves leading from them [the vertebrae] will disturb the organs to which they run.'

Cullen's nerve flow concept and Harrison's choice of spinal manipulation were taken on board by J. Evans Riadore when he wrote *Irritation of the Spinal Nerves* in 1843, two years before D.D. Palmer was born. According to Riadore: 'If any organ is deficiently supplied with nervous energy or of blood, its functions immediately, and sooner or later its structure become deranged,' and he advised manipulation as the preferred method of correction. One year before Palmer's first adjustment on Harvey Lillard, the prominent London physician Sir William Gowers underlined the importance of the nervous system in disease when he stated, 'Function depends on the release of force

– nerve force.' Those words sound so familiar that they might well have come from the lips of Daniel David Palmer himself.

NERVE IMPINGEMENT AND THE SUBLUXATION

Palmer renamed Cullen's vital nerve force of *vis medicatrix naturae* 'Innate Intelligence', and believed that it derived from God, whom he called 'Universal Intelligence'. He held that Innate was stored in the brain and that it flowed through the spinal cord and out through the nerves to reach every organ and tissue of the body. The flow of Innate could be interrupted by the impingement, or stretching, of the nerve against the vertebrae as it left the spine. This process of impingement was induced by vertebral subluxation – or malpositioning – and went on to increase or decrease the body's 'tone' (nerve tension) to create disease. He held that:

> 95 per cent of all diseases are the result of slightly displaced vertebrae which press against nerves causing impingements, the result being too much or not enough functioning, and the other 5 per cent are from luxated joints elsewhere than in the spinal column.

Health was harmony, as represented by a stringed instrument. When tone was increased the pitch was higher, as in a violin string drawn too tight, and when it was decreased the slackened string produced a lower note. Faulty tone led to dis-harmony or, as Palmer termed it, 'dis-ease'. The subluxations which, through impingement, disrupted tone were induced by accidents, toxins, or by auto-suggestion. Adjustment of the subluxated joint was followed by a recovery period as the flow of Innate was restored and the body was thereby empowered to return itself to full health. Needless to say, health would only be maintained so long as the subluxation's causative factors were kept at bay.

NERVE COMPRESSION AND THE SUBLUXATION

B.J. Palmer challenged his father's hypothesis that a nerve could be stretched, and asserted that Innate Intelligence was disrupted by 'compression', or direct pressure on the nerve by the displaced vertebra. Although there was vehement disagreement over the exact process, all early chiropractors believed that disease resulted from nerve disruption by subluxations. As a term, subluxation came to include not only minor displacements of joints, but any mechanical malfunction, together with the neurological symptoms that followed. The spinal subluxation theory clearly differentiated early chiropractors from early osteopaths, who believed that disease was caused by what they termed spinal lesions resulting from interrupted blood supply to the spinal cord, nerves, and tissues.

MERIC SYSTEM

Physiologists by the end of the last century had already started mapping out the autonomic nervous system, which controls all our subconscious bodily functions such as digestion, heart rate, hormonal balances, and tissue repair. Their published work identified the nerve pathways, or links, between the spinal cord – protected by its ring of spinal bones and joints – the sympathetic ganglia lying in front of the vertebrae, and the body's organs at the end of the line. It was argued by the chiropractors that the dramatic cures they were achieving for all manner of diseases could be explained by the adjustment's restoration of nerve flow along these pathways, from spinal cord to organ via the sympathetic ganglia. Using these physiological maps it was now possible to link the organs to specific 'zones' or 'planes' of vertebral nerve supply. A patient complaining of heart disease would therefore be suffering from a subluxation at one of the levels supplying the heart and particular attention would then be paid to the Heart Place in the region of the second Thoracic vertebra. Indigestion would be linked to a subluxation of the sixth, seventh, or eighth Thoracic, site of the Stomach Place. There would be an attempt to 'nerve trace' tenderness from one of the suspected vertebrae which, when found, would invite a specific adjustment. The resulting restoration of nerve function then allowed the body to start healing itself as intended by nature.

This theory differed little from the published works on *Spinal Irritation* of Dr Isaac Parrish in the 1830s, from the 1894 statement on nerve force by Sir William Gowers, and from the manipulative remedies chosen by Edward Harrison and J. Evans Riadore, yet by the twentieth century this mechanism was hotly denounced by established medicine as quackery. In spite of this ridicule there were proven links, and in 1934 the noted ortho-paedic surgeon Joel Goldthwait acknowledged the presence of 'pathology and functional disturbance due to mechanical causes, usually the result of pressure or stretching of the nerve roots'. Although he went on to state that interference to the nerve roots produced referred pain which only imitated organ pain, he acknowledged that chiropractic adjustment corrected the spinal lesion and removed the symptoms. However, by the time of Goldthwait's pronouncement, B.J. Palmer had already taken his branch of chiropractic way beyond the pale of scientific acceptance by evolving a theory that disease was to be cured only by adjusting the upper cervical vertebrae.

HOLE-IN-ONE

Both Palmers had regarded the brain as the seat of Innate Intelligence, which then communicated with every cell of the body through Mental Impulses passing along the nerves. As the brainstem descends into the upper cervical vertebrae, B.J. regarded it as a site of special significance. Soon he was teaching that it was subluxations of the first three vertebrae leading from the skull that preceded all others, and that it was here that specific adjustment would gain a quick and lasting response. As the introducer of radiography to the chiropractic profession it was only natural that he should devise an intricate system of X-ray analysis for the occiput and upper cervical spine using careful measurement to identify the 'major' subluxation.

He accepted that other subluxations existed but held that these could only be secondary to the major and would recur until the major had been corrected by specific adjustment. His X-ray measurement indicated the 'line of drive', or direction, of the adjustment. Its mode of delivery was through his toggle recoil. This is an exceptionally rapid adjustment designed for its directional accuracy, speed, comfort, and efficacy, and it evolved in response to a call for the additional directional specificity demanded by this technique.

Although the analysis and execution of B.J.'s new approach was complex, the theory which accompanied it was not. He referred to the Garden Hose or Dynamo Theory, and likened the compression of the spinal cord to a kink in a garden hose. Flow of mental impulses would remain sluggish so long as the subluxation remained, but as normal flow is restored to the hose when the kink is removed, so correction of the subluxation by adjustment removes nerve pressure, restoring the flow of mental impulses to the system. Likewise, any interference with the flow of electricity from a dynamo will lessen the power received at its destination, dimming the light-bulb. Remove the interference and power is restored. Full health follows.

Palmer's correction of the major subluxation with one adjustment led to the coinage of the term 'Hole-In-One' (H.I.O.), not only for its parallel with that rare and great golfing accomplishment but because of the graphic relationship of atlas and axis. The Hole is represented by the circular atlas (first vertebra). This is impaled by the dens of the axis (second vertebra) which, when viewed from the side, represents the figure One. Held by Palmer to be the peak of chiropractic's development, graduates of the Palmer School were imbued with the merits of H.I.O. from the 1930s to the mid-1950s, to the exclusion of all other techniques. The Palmer School became increasingly isolated as a result, driving a wedge of opinion through the heart of the chiropractic profession. Finally the faculty rebelled and recommended the reintroduction of full spinal adjusting. This met with reluctant approval from Palmer when he granted his assent in 1957, and the following year marked the beginning of the end for the exclusive use of the Hole-in-One technique. Shortly after this, adjustment of non-spinal joints was added to the curriculum so that now all the joints of the body could again be tackled. Writing on chiropractic theories in 1980, Robert A. Leach estimated that fewer than 5 per cent of the profession exclusively used H.I.O. technique then, and that figure must be less than 3 per cent today.

BONE OUT OF PLACE THEORY

Bonesetters were named, not because they reset broken bones, but because it was thought their manipulations set displaced bones back into place. Following in the footsteps of bonesetters it is understandable that both chiropractors and osteopaths should accept this theory, the chiropractor visualizing misplaced bones compressing the nerve, while the osteopath envisaged interruption to the blood flow.

Chiropractors believed that any vertebral misalignment would alter the shape of the intervertebral foramen, the bony arch through which the spinal nerve leaves the spinal column. Because the foramen is formed by two adjacent vertebrae, and one is capable of becoming misplaced against the other, any resultant mechanical pressure would impinge (cause stretching) on the nerve. D.D. Palmer's impingement theory was opposed by his son, who taught that misplaced vertebrae would compress the nerve, and B.J. would later assert that this compression occurred between the base of the skull and the first three vertebrae, interfering with the brainstem.

The vertebral misalignment theory was particularly acceptable to most chiropractors, not only because it explained their nerve irritation hypothesis, but because they believed the evidence could be seen on X-ray. In theory, the offending vertebrae might be shown tilting or rotating to one side or the other before the adjustment. After treatment a repeat X-ray would, it was believed, demonstrate the return of the vertebrae to their normal or near-normal positions. The theory gave rise to a number of highly specific adjustment techniques designed to re-place the vertebra by thrusting in precisely the direction indicated by the X-ray.

DISC OUT OF PLACE THEORY

The advent of spinal surgery drew attention to the role of the intervertebral disc in many cases of severe spinal pain referring into the arm or leg. In such cases the centre of the disc was seen to be bulging through a crack in its outer lining, whereupon it drove the nerve root against solid vertebral bone. Removal of the disc or its bulging nucleus by the surgeon released nerve pressure, so that in many cases pain subsided altogether. There was therefore a tendency in orthopaedic and manipulative medicine to look at the majority of back problems as being related to various degrees of disc bulge, and more attention was applied to those manipulative techniques which rotate the spine, theoretically stretching taut the anulus (criss-cross fibrous outer lining) to create a vacuum that would suck the disc bulge back in.

Such emphasis led to the 'slipped disc' being made responsible for almost every manifestation of spinal pain, and although the disc can neither slip in or out it became a popular label for all to use, doctor and patient alike.

MODIFIED PRESSURE THEORY

The theories of compression run into difficulties when the composition of the intervertebral foramen is examined. The foramen is the bony canal that carries the nerve from the spinal cord and out of the vertebral column, and it is here that many cases of compression occur. However, the nerve itself occupies only 30 to 50 per cent of the threatened area and the remainder is made up of an artery, a vein, lymph vessels, fibrous tissues, the small recurrent meningeal nerve, and an infilling of fat. In order to effectively compress a nerve, a subluxation would have to be massive. Clearly some other mechanism must be at work to allow quite small subluxations to manifest themselves.

Writing from his native Switzerland in 1938, chiropractor Fred Illi emphasized the importance of the recurrent meningeal nerve. The spine is made up of segments which correspond to each of the vertebrae. Each segment produces a nerve root to carry the spinal nerve away from the cord and through the foramen. The recurrent nerve is a branch of the spinal nerve and it returns through the foramen to regulate the blood flow that nourishes its own original segment. In this way Illi argued: 'Every segment of the spinal cord controls its own nourishment through the action of a short reflex arc which may be called a self supporting mechanism.'

Irritation of the recurrent nerve would either induce a flooding of blood vessels with consequent tissue engorgement and in-direct nerve pressure, or, in rarer cases, a constriction of blood supply to the spinal cord segment and nerves associated with it. Both mechanisms lead to the constellation of signs and symptoms recognized by chiropractors as indicative of a subluxation, and through removing recurrent nerve irritation by adjustment these would disappear. Illi believed that quite small subluxations would be sufficient to irritate the recurrent meningeal nerve.

THE CHIROPRACTIC FIXATION CONCEPT

In placing great emphasis on the importance of X-rays and the relative position of vertebrae, chiropractors tended to fall into the trap of viewing the spine as they saw it on X-ray. By adjusting the vertebra that was shown to be 'out of place' they were able to restore its position, so that if the patient was X-rayed again that vertebra would now be shown 'back in line'.

The spine was usually examined from a purely static point of view in the manner it appeared on an X-ray plate. There had never been a need to equate the out of place vertebra with any abnormal movement that might accompany it. This was to change with the work of Henri Gillet. Unable to gain access to spinal X-rays in his native Belgium, where chiropractic was and still is illegal, Gillet began to concentrate on devising methods of vertebral measurement in the 1930s, later incorporating his findings with those of others in *Belgian Chiropractic Research Notes*. His methods regard the spine as a series of mobile units so that alterations of normal movement as detected by hand can then be equated with the subluxation.

While Gillet was developing his system of 'motion palpation' in chiropractic, medical researchers Schmorl and Junghans started to emphasize the function of the vertebral joint as a unit made up of many parts. Working in the 1950s they served to draw the attention of research away from merely those structures appearing on X-ray, directing it instead towards all the components that make up a living, moving, spinal joint. Their vertebral motor unit, as they termed it, was composed not only of bone and disc but included ligaments, muscles, blood vessels, joint capsules, nerves, fluids, and supporting tissues – each with a role to play in the function of the unit, which is primarily one of movement. Researchers now began to study the mechanisms of spinal movement as a whole and how these could be disrupted.

Probably the first reference to motion analysis in chiropractic literature is that of the Dane, Henning Hviid, in 1955. As a student at the Danish School of Chiropractic, Hviid had been influenced by Finn Christensen, who in his turn had absorbed the writings of Lewis and Kellgren and of Inman and Saunders during the 1940s. Each area of the spine, whether it be the neck, thorax, or lower back, has a specific range of movement within which every one of its vertebrae plays a part. Should one of these vertebrae become fixed to its neighbour, the adjoining joints must necessarily compensate for this restriction by increasing their own movements. In time this additional work will overload the small muscles, ligaments, and joint capsules involved in compensatory activity. Repetitive strains induce pain and then contraction in surrounding muscles, returning as a vicious cycle, fixing the area even more forcefully, increasing local pain and inflammation, and producing 'referred pain' patterns that are felt in distant areas.

Hviid quoted the work of Lewis and Kellgren, whose injections of salt water between vertebrae had induced autonomic reactions such as raised blood pressure. He went on to suggest that vertebral irritation from malfunctions of the motor unit could lead to autonomic symptoms, and that the vicious cycle could be broken by chiropractic adjustment, restoring full movement and eliminating the symptoms.

Hviid attributed the initial fixing of a vertebral unit to muscle tension induced by irritants such as minor displacements, other fixed vertebrae, strains, poor posture, draughts, cold, and psychological factors. Gillet later included certain dietary irritants in his list of causative factors. Both recognized the importance of the autonomic reflexes which link the spinal musculature to the smooth visceral muscle of the body's internal organs, so that when the adjustment instantaneously releases the spinal muscle, its visceral counterpart follows suit. 'Surely this is the explanation of the curing of diseases such as bronchial asthma, dysmenorrhoea, and spasmodic intestinal attacks,' said Hviid.

During the 1960s there was a gradual acceptance by the European chiropractic profession that the old theories of nerve pressure and vertebral misalignment were no longer viable. Not only was modern physiological research beginning to challenge old chiropractic mechanisms, but the concept of the chiropractic fixation was becoming more widely acepted. In the United States, Homewood's classic book, *The Neurodynamics of the Vertebral Subluxation*, published in 1962, was probably the spur, for one of his classifications of subluxation was based upon the disruption of normal vertebral movement by fixation. Since that time, chiropractic literature the world over has increasingly accepted the fixation pattern as one of major importance. The joint is fixed within its normal range of motion, usually irregularly, in which case it appears on X-ray as the 'odd-one-out'. When the joint locks in the neutral resting position X-ray evidence is less helpful. The fixation is always accompanied by changes in the surrounding soft tissues, by lessened mobility, and by altered local pain patterns. Occasionally it disrupts normal neurological action to induce referred pain or autonomic disturbances. The work started by Gillet in Belgium has now been championed by Leonard Faye's Motion Palpation Institute in the United States, and is now almost universally accepted by chiropractic colleges the world over as explaining the mechanism of spinal dysfunction.

VERTEBRAL HYPERMOBILITY

Vertebral fixation restricts movement which must now occur elsewhere if overall mobility is not to be lost. Such compensatory movement can overload a neighbouring joint introducing excessive mobility (hypermobility) and strain either above or below the fixation. Sometimes these strains can occur in the absence of a fixation, particularly if one of the common structural anomalies is present, or if a patient's posture or working position overloads a series of vertebrae. Once a vertebral joint has become unstable and excessively mobile the problem will often worsen, for joints above or below become lazy and cease to move fully. There is no need for them to move if all movement is already being taken up in the hypermobile joint, and their stiffening serves to compound the problem. Consequently, the ligaments that normally restrain the joint will lengthen, the disc and one or both facets begin to wear through overwork, and the early degenerative changes of osteoarthritis (called spondylosis on the spine) begin to take effect. The inflammatory changes that accompany this process not only cause pain locally but, as with fixations, can trigger referred pain and stimulate autonomic reflexes to induce internal organ malfunction.

The chiropractic adjustment is normally directed at mobilizing the stiff neighbouring areas, but a rapid shallow stretch of the hypermobile joint is occasionally called for to induce a reflex reaction, contracting the slack over-lengthened vertebral muscles and thereby tightening the joint. Almost all cases of vertebral hypermobility need follow-up treatment, corrective exercises, changes in posture, or other preventive measures. The importance of X-rays to identify one of the common abnormalities of bone structure that frequently accompany the hypermobility syndrome cannot be overemphasized.

THE AUTONOMIC REFLEXES

Since its early years the chiropractic profession has looked on the autonomic nervous system as the mechanism through which adjustments influence the internal body organs, and the Meric System was devised in rather a cook-book fashion to link individual organs to specific vertebrae. As the sum of scientific knowledge grew through the twentieth century it became rather more easy for medical adversaries to pick holes in such simplistic explanations.

Having closer links with the medical mainstream, American osteopathic researchers were able to gain support and funding for studies into the effects of vertebral lesions on the autonomic nervous system, and their first results were published as early as 1907. Their first animal experiments demonstrated that inter-vertebral lesions could influence blood supply to prompt changes in urine production, intestinal movement, gastric secretion, blood plasma pigments, endocrine secretion, and lung function.

Later osteopathic, medical, and chiropractic research has indicated that spinal subluxations can stimulate somato-autonomic reflexes (those nerve connections between areas under our conscious control, such as a vertebral joint, and areas out of our normal control, such as one of the internal visceral organs). These reflexes can in turn disrupt normal bodily functions. It is this mechanism that chiropractors turn to in order to explain many of the referred pain patterns, muscular wasting, asthma, bronchitis, collapsed lung, spasm of coronary arteries, painful periods, gastric complaints, and intestinal disorders.

The somato-autonomic reflexes provide the most logical explanation for the success of chiropractic adjustment in correcting many visceral disorders. Those in the medical profession who have devoted time and patience in developing manipulative skills beyond normal orthopaedic levels agree. The Canadian orthopaedic specialist J.F. Bourdillon refers to such conditions as 'reflex sympathetic dystrophy', linking spinal joint subluxations to such symptoms as excessive sweating, water retention, bone wasting, skin circulation changes, wrist or ankle swelling, carpal tunnel syndrome, painful heels, and flat feet. He is even prepared to describe a case of deafness which he cured by spinal manipulation at the thoracic level, emulating that first adjustment by D.D. Palmer on Harvey Lillard, and although he admitted the exact mechanism remained unclear to him he attributed it to autonomic involvement.

In the United States one of the most respected figures in manual medicine, John Mennell, explained:

> Pain from joint pathology may be appreciated in any distant structure which shares its nerve supply with the joint. Indeed, one may postulate interference with the function of viscera as a result of referred joint pain through a somatic/visceral reflex arc. I am certain that such phenomena occur.

In Britain physiotherapist Gregory Grieve developed his skills into advanced manipulative therapy and went on to recount how numerous examples of migraine, vertigo, visual disturbances, hearing impairment, and respiratory and abdominal problems can be related by 'all those experienced in manipulation'.

In West Germany, with a developed manual medicine tradition, numerous researchers have accounted for their success in treating visceral problems with manipulation through this mechansim. Influenced by early chiropractors, prominent medical professors established the Society for the Research and Development of Chirotherapy (FAC). One senior professor, K. Gutzeit, described spinal subluxation as the 'initiator, provocator, multiplacator, and localisator' of many organic diseases. His student, Professor Werner Kunert, later went on to explain the many pathways within the somato-autonomic system that are involved, and asserted: 'There can, in fact, be no doubt that the state of the spinal column does have a bearing on the functional status of the internal organs.'

In Eastern bloc countries manipulative treatment has been able to develop unthwarted within the medical system. Czech neurologist Dr Karel Lewit accepts that a painful stimulus to a spinal segment induces a somatic response (local muscle spasm and restricted mobility at the vertebral joint) and in addition an autonomic response which is 'much more varied'. This varied response can be local and may involve spinal blood flow reduction, numbness, and pain spots. It can also show central effects that 'may affect respiration, and the cardiovascular or the digestive systems'. Introduced to chiropractic by a Palmer-trained chiropractor from his native land, Lewit's published work describes the success he has experienced in using manipulation to treat cases of tonsillitis, breathing problems, heart disease, digestive conditions, gynaecological disorders, migraine, vertigo, dizziness, and other illnesses.

It is clear that chiropractors' use of the autonomic reflexes to explain their daily successes in treating organic conditions has been amply backed up by those in the medical profession who have been able to develop skills in advanced spinal manual diagnosis and treatment. However, as with a very great deal in medicine, this mechanism is not actually proven clinically and therefore remains just a working hypothesis to explain that success. Further clinical research must be forthcoming if chiropractors are to justify their treatment of organic complaints on a regular basis. Until then chiropractors will primarily be associated with the treatment of musculo-skeletal complaints and some types of headache, with are more readily proven. This should not preclude them from treating carefully selected organic problems where a demonstrable vertebral connection exists, for although medical antagonists have scorned Palmer's successful restoration of Harvey Lillard's hearing for over ninety years, there are now highly-respected members of the medical profession who have shared that experience with the 'Discoverer of Chiropractic'.

CEREBRAL BLOOD FLOW THEORY

Chiropractic adjustment often relieves various types of head-ache, including the migraine type commonly associated with altered blood flow to the brain. Other symptoms such as tinnitus, vertigo, nausea, and dizziness may also respond. Medical and chiropractic authorities have linked these symptoms to auto-nomic disturbances which induce spasm of the vertebral artery to the brain, altering blood flow. There are others who hold that blood supply to the brain can be disturbed by subluxations in the neck that deflect or compress the vertebral arteries as they pass up through the cervical vertebrae, loop over the atlas vertebra, and enter the brain cavity of the skull to supply the brainstem.

Many patients suffer such symptoms later in life, and here it is thought that the bony outgrowths that accompany cervical spondylosis (arthritis of the neck) are responsible. If a chiropractor suspects vertebral artery involvement he or she will perform tests to rule out any risks from conventional manipulation. If any doubt exists, a non-force technique such as the 'Activator' or one of the soft-tissue methods is sure to be employed.

NEUROGENIC HEAD PAIN THEORY

The work of Nikolai Bogduk in Australia, and other medical researchers during the 1980s, has called into question the cerebral blood flow theory which has been in vogue for some sixty years. Bogduk found that by selectively anaesthetizing the cervical facet joints he was able to banish pain that was referred elsewhere, so that lower neck, shoulder, and chest pain responded to anaesthesis of facet joints in the lower neck, whilst anaesthesis of upper neck facets removed head pain.

He has postulated that as the first three cervical nerves receive branches from joints and ligaments in this region their activation by faulty joint mechanics has repercussions elsewhere. These nerves converge centrally with the spinal nucleus of the trigeminal nerve which in turn stimulates a part of the brainstem called the locus ceruleus. This structure has been shown upon stimulation to raise blood pressure, to constrict the Internal and dilate the External Carotid arteries, and thereby to induce headache or migrainous pain.

Once again medical science has come to the aid of chiropractic, showing that the profession has nothing to fear from serious research. Where a chiropractic technique works so demonstrably in practice there must always be a rational explanation as to why.

SUBLUXATION STRESS THEORY

D.D. Palmer claimed that variations in nerve tone meant the difference between good health and disease and that subluxations adversely affected nerve tone. A number of chiropractors over the past thirty years have taken this a step further, claiming that nerve tone can be equated with the level of stress within the nervous system. In the 1950s Dr Hans Selye demonstrated to the scientific community the link between stressful stimuli and the neuro-endocrine and immune systems. This led to a recognition of the role that chronic psychological stress factors play in the disease process, so much so that medical practitioners in the 1960s, 1970s and 1980s prescribed sedatives indiscriminately for almost any condition. There can be little doubt that undue stress causes breakdown in the immune system by acting through the nervous and endocrine systems. Chiropractors argue that a chronic vertebral fixation or subluxation is a potent stress factor that bombards the nervous system with irritating stimuli, setting up immune system deficiency. Elimination of this constant stress factor through the successful adjustment of the subluxation allows the body to regain its natural resistance to disease.

MODERN ATTITUDES

Throughout the world chiropractic training today encourages a questioning attitude in young chiropractors. The blind faith that served to strengthen the resolve of chiropractors in those difficult years of ridicule and legal persecution has been replaced by a confidence based upon sound knowledge and learning. Chiropractic has gained a respect within the world at large that enables it to cross professional barriers with ease. Chiropractors are now important contributors at every major symposium on spinal pain. After attending the 1987 International Chiropractic Conference in London a senior British spinal surgeon, Alan Gardner, told the assembly: 'This has been one of the most impressive spinal programmes I have ever attended.' Canadian professor of orthopaedics, William Kirkaldy-Willis wrote:

> I never thought that in my lifetime I would see such happy co-operation between chiropractors and orthopaedic surgeons. I found the same new outlook during a recent visit to Finland, and at the 'Challenge of the Lumbar Spine' Symposium recently in New York. It is so very exciting that in the future we shall all be able to work together.

Chapter 9

CHIROPRACTIC TECHNIQUES

I created the art of adjusting vertebrae, using the spinous and transverse processes as levers, and named the mental act of accumulating knowledge . . . together with the science, art and philosophy – chiropractic. *Daniel D. Palmer* (1845–1913)

The manipulative techniques described by the Hippocratic Corpus and by Galen remained relatively unchanged until the late nineteenth century, as illustrations of the French surgeon Calot have shown. The principle of using assistants to traction the patient while the physician applied pressure dominated the orthodox medical approach, although bonesetters world-wide had evolved less dramatic methods. These usually involved stretching the offending area until a joint 'crack' could be heard, whereupon the bone would be 'set' back in place. Early osteopathic techniques are very closely based on such generalized stretching movements and clearly follow the bonesetting tradition.

SPECIFICITY

It was Palmer's insistence on a specific contact directly upon the spinous or transverse process, using these as levers, which set chiropractic apart. Chiropractors began from the start to concentrate on refining their adjustments in order to determine the exact direction and precise depth of thrust required for a specific vertebral movement. From these earliest days the quest has been to develop more and more refined forms of adjustment, so that the manipulative action concentrates on moving one joint, and one joint alone, in a predetermined direction and with a predetermined force.

As osteopathy and chiropractic developed along their individual paths, chiropractors distanced themselves from their cousins by emphasizing what they called their specific adjustment and by contrasting it with the osteopathic long lever techniques, which usually involved the stretching of several joints at a time. Early osteopaths developed generalized lengthy rocking and stretching movements over a wide area, which they called articulation. Chiropractors dissociated themselves from articulation, although Henri Gillet's Motion Palpation examination techniques involve similar rocking movements which Gillet acknowledges have a beneficial articulatory effect. This examination method is now being used more and more widely the world over, especially in Europe, and it could be argued that articulation has entered the realms of chiropractic treatment unheralded and through the back door.

ANALYSIS

The chiropractic emphasis on specificity not only calls for adjustment techniques that are exact and precise, but systems of analysis to identify those joints which are at fault. Early chiropractic methods relied upon observation and touch. Noting of obvious deformities such as a deviated spinous process, short leg, rotated pelvis, prominent rib, or tilted skull would be followed by observation of the skin for colour changes, and then by palpation. Using touch, the chiropractor would note changes in temperature, feel the resilience of the surrounding tissues, and localize areas of tenderness. Much emphasis in the early years was placed on nerve tracing – following a line of tenderness from the vertebra along the course of an associated nerve – although this has now been largely abandoned.

Following techniques devised by Henri Gillet and others, nowadays, greater emphasis is placed upon motion palpation. This involves taking each joint through its varied ranges of motion to determine whether it moves too much or too little, and in which direction. In other words, modern chiropractors have ceased to examine the spine solely in its resting state, and now localize with motion palpation those functions of movement which it fails to perform correctly.

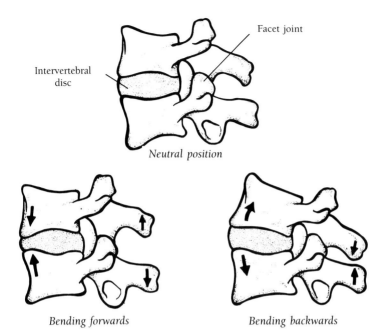

Neutral position

Bending forwards   *Bending backwards*

Vertebrae in motion (side view). On bending forwards and backwards one part of the disc is compressed and another stretched. Backward bending forces the facet joint surfaces together, whilst forward bending separates them. Individual vertebrae may lock in any of these, or other positions, including the neutral position. Chiropractic adjustment will release the joints, allowing normal movement to be restored

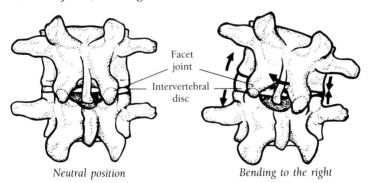

Neutral position   *Bending to the right*

Vertebrae in motion (back view). On bending to the right the disc and facet joints are compressed on the right and stretched apart on the left. Vertebrae may lock in this (or any other) position. Chiropractic adjustment will release the joints, allowing normal movement to be restored

In the quest for greater specificity B.J. Palmer devised instruments such as the neurocalometer to detect hot or cold spots, and others used electricity (as galvanic current) to identify areas of increased sweat gland activity, one of the autonomic reactions. As with most gimmicks few instruments have survived, and some chiropractors condemned them as being contrary to chiropractic principles for such analysis is clearly not 'done by hand'. Philosophical argument apart, the real test is whether they uncover important factors not detectable by hand that would enable the chiropractor to succeed where others had failed. No instrument has regularly passed this test, leading every one of them to follow the path of obsolescence. Every one, that is, except the X-ray unit, and that was introduced into the Palmer School in 1910 amidst great controversy.

X-RAY ANALYSIS

Unable to accept on philosophical grounds the pioneering X-ray work begun by B.J. Palmer, Joy M. Loban defected to form the Universal College. 'One morning, in mid-April 1910, as if by prearranged signal, forty or fifty of the students arose and marched out of the classroom, down the hill to Brady and Sixth Streets, and the next thing everybody knew a new school of chiropractic was in operation in Davenport,' recounted A. August Dye. Nevertheless, X-ray analysis was no flash in the pan, and was to grow to become the hallmark of chiropractic's search for specificity. It is ironic that the first standing X-rays, preferred by most chiropractors for recording gravitational influences, were taken at Universal College in 1918, showing that even such heart-felt convictions, born under such emotive circumstances, will succumb to an outcome that consistently benefits the patient. A recent study shows that 81 per cent of British chiropractors have on site X-ray installations, and their code of practice demands that the remainder must have local facilities available to enable radiographic studies to be made whenever necessary. In the Canadian province of Ontario, with over 1,000 chiropractors, two out of every three have their own facilities.

X-rays not only help a chiropractor to understand exactly what is wrong with a patient, but may also throw light on why it has happened and how far the problem has progressed. They help rule out bone disease and enable the chiropractor to estimate the chances of success with a particular problem. They are valuable in patient re-education, assisting patients to visualize their own specific problem, and by providing detail on the direction of individual joint surfaces (which differ from patient to patient) they help the chiropractor choose the most comfortable and effective specific adjustment for that patient. In sworn testimony before the New Zealand Government Commission of Inquiry into Chiropractic, Dr Scott Haldeman, medical neurologist and chiropractor, stated of chiropractors: 'If they give their manipulation, their adjustment, in a direction indicated from the X-ray, then they are likely to be able to give the adjustment with less force, less dramatically, less painfully and with better effect than if they do not use the X-ray.'

During the 1950s, 1960s, and 1970s, a number of treatment systems developed around the detailed measurement of land-marks on an X-ray plate. The most successful were those developed by Gonstead, Pettibon, and Grostic, but with chiro-practic colleges placing a greater emphasis on concepts of vertebral motion, these techniques cease to be as popular today.

LABORATORY ANALYSIS

Modern chiropractic colleges teach the taking and analysing of blood and urine samples. Although the majority of chiropractors do not possess their own laboratory facilities they refer their patients for the appropriate tests when this is called for. The actual analysis is unlikely to help with the specificity of an adjustment, but it may reveal conditions that require referral elsewhere or factors which might limit the choice of adjustment to a non-force technique.

RANGE OF TECHNIQUES

Chiropractic methods range from classical adjustments, where the thrust is applied to a contact on the structure to be moved, through to indirect thrust techniques with the contact point elsewhere. In addition there are techniques which are applied not to the solid structures around the joint but to the muscles and ligaments, or soft tissues of that joint, and there are general loosening or mobilizing techniques. Some of the soft tissue mobilizing techniques used by chiropractors today have been gleaned from other manual therapies such as remedial massage, physical therapy, naturopathy, and osteopathy, and many chiropractors regard them as useful adjuncts to prepare the ground for their chiropractic adjustment, or to enhance its effects. Hot and cold therapies are fairly widely used, and in recent years some chiropractors have added physiotherapy equipment to their armoury. The most popular methods are ultrasound and short-wave diathermy, and most chiropractic colleges introduced a physical therapy curriculum when the subject became an elective part of the United States National Board of Chiropractic Examiners diploma. Chiropractors have generally taken care not to fall into the same trap as physio-therapists – neglecting the manual approach in favour of treating several patients at a time with pre-set machines. By using hands rather than instruments chiropractors can respond rapidly and accurately to soft tissues as they relax, varying their therapeutic movements the instant the body responds.

DIRECT THRUST TECHNIQUES

Direct techniques, such as those used by D.D. Palmer to lever the spinous or transverse processes, form the core of chiropractic. These are classically 'high velocity thrusts', with a carefully measured force rapidly applied. Actual joint movement is minimal, and any slack within the joint must be removed during the build-up to the adjustment. Movement must be sufficient to carry the joint beyond its voluntary range, whilst remaining within that range permitted by nature. Very often there is a joint crack, which researchers at Leeds University have identified as a vacuum-created nitrogen bubble bursting within the joint as a result of rapid joint stretch. Adjustment should normally be quite painless, although firm pressure applied beforehand on a recently inflamed joint may sometimes create temporary dis-comfort. The secrets of a painless adjustment are removal of joint slack to prevent it from bouncing back and an accurate line of drive (direction of thrust). Slack is removed as the patient relaxes enough to allow the chiropractor to take the joint to its full range of comfortable movement, and then it is adjusted away from any pain-provoking direction along that line of drive which will most successfully separate the two joint surfaces. Usually the line of

Ranges of movement

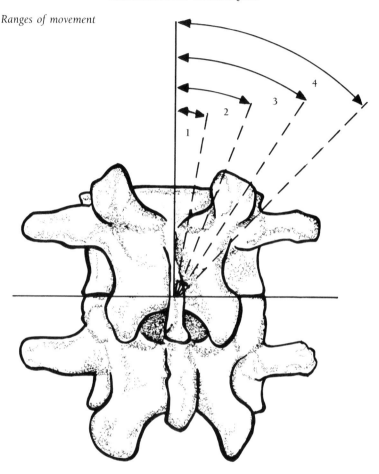

1 Range of movement in a restricted joint

2 Range of voluntary movement in a normal joint

3 Range to which a joint will move when passively stretched. It's limit is termed the *Elastic barrier of resistance*. Physiotherapy mobilizing techniques do not exceed this

4 Full anatomic range of movement in a normal joint. Chiropractic adjustment goes beyond the *Elastic barrier of resistance* but never beyond the anatomic range

drive can be determined by palpation and a detailed knowledge of that joint's anatomy, but X-rays enable the chiropractor to take into consideration such commonly found anomalies as irregu-

171

larly shaped facet joints, making the chiropractic adjustment less likely to provoke discomfort than other methods.

At times circumstances determine the choice of slower stretching adjustments, which can be facilitated by releasing sections of a specially designed chiropractic couch. Various forms of manually applied traction may also be applied if circumstances call for this approach, and a few chiropractors possess mechanical traction devices.

INDIRECT THRUST TECHNIQUES

Indirect techniques involve using a pad, towel, or wedge to gently stretch a joint. The pad might be used to act as a fulcrum

Toggle recoil adjustment

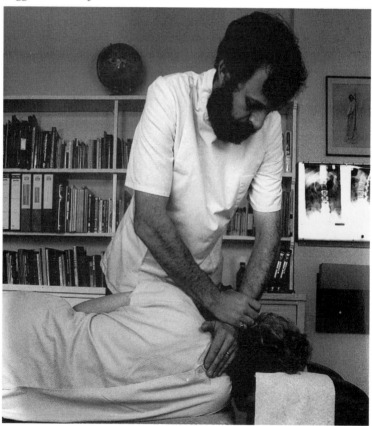

while a joint is carefully opened over it. Several techniques have been devised for adjusting the sacro-iliac joints using wedge-shaped blocks placed at different points of the pelvis, so that the patient's own body weight gently opens the locked joint. This method is particularly valuable when traditional methods might cause discomfort, although several minutes must pass for it to take effect instead of the split second response of a normal adjustment.

SOFT TISSUE TECHNIQUES

Soft tissue techniques may be used to prepare a joint for adjustment, to help remove joint slack, to enhance the effects of an adjustment, or as techniques devised in their own right to free a joint, create a permanent muscle relaxation response, or trigger a neurological reaction. Methods range from simple muscle stretching, standard remedial massage, 'trigger-point' pressure, muscle 'goading', and 'reciprocal innervation' techniques. A method for provoking trigger-points devised by Raymond Nimmo is described later (p. 178), but goading techniques are used to provoke weak muscles into activity, whilst reciprocal innervation methods involve the patient stretching a muscle against resistance to bring about a neurological response that will, on completion, relax that muscle and restore greater movement.

MOBILIZING TECHNIQUES

Certain conditions call for techniques that will take a joint or series of joints through a full range of repeated movements that are designed to increase mobility. They may be passive, when the patient relaxes as he or she is carried through these movements by the chiropractor, or they may be active, when the manoeuvres are performed by the patient. Often a patient will be given specific active mobilizing exercises to practise at home.

TOGGLE RECOIL ADJUSTMENT

The first twenty years of chiropractic development saw D.D. Palmer's leverage techniques on the spinous and transverse processes refined, but left relatively unchanged. However, his son B.J., ever determined to leave his individual imprint, introduced his Toggle Recoil technique. In mechanical terms a toggle consists of two elbow or knee-like joints at East and West with their shafts connected to each other at North and South. When East and West are drawn together North and South are driven apart. In such an adjustment the upper torso forms the Northern component whilst the wrists interlock to form the Southern part. East and West are represented by the elbows. As the elbows straighten rapidly the forearms are brought together and the wrist contact drives down in a measured specific direction. The movement is so rapid that the contact is maintained for only a split second, recoiling away as the maximum depth is reached. This technique proved faster, more accurate, and more controllable than any other technique devised at that time, and it was so different in appearance from all others that many consider it peculiarly chiropractic. It became the trademark of its inventor B.J. Palmer, along with his neurocalometer. In the 1930s, 1940s and 1950s it was the only method taught to B.J.'s Straight chiropractors, and was applied as the Upper Cervical Specific technique or Hole-in-One. Although still an important part of a modern chiropractor's training, probably fewer than 3 per cent use it exclusively today, preferring to pick and choose the most appropriate method from the massive armoury of techniques now available.

In England, almost as if in a time-warp, a modified version of B.J. Palmer's toggle recoil has evolved as a therapy in its own

Spinous hook rotary lumbar adjustment

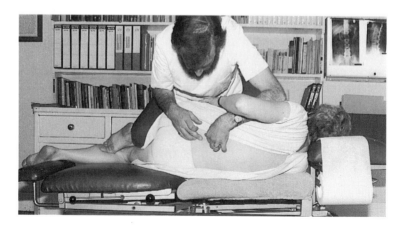

right. Adapted in the late 1940s by patient John McTimoney from his personal experience of chiropractic treatment, this method has been taught as a part-time home study course in Oxfordshire since 1972. After his death in 1981 his 14 followers mushroomed to a group of over one hundred by 1989, and grouping themselves as the Institute of Pure Chiropractic they strive to preserve what they perceive as D.D. Palmer's 'original technique that was lost'. By contrast, the vast majority of chiropractors are not tied to any one technique and are therefore able to select the most appropriate method available, including the Toggle Recoil, to elicit the mechanical and neurological effects required in the patient.

ROTATION METHODS

Rotary techniques are directly-applied thrusts that involve twisting the joint round through its natural range of movement in order to remove any slackness. These are commonly applied to the neck or lower back, and may be performed sitting or lying on the back, side, or front. Before applying a rotary adjustment to the neck the chiropractor will normally undertake a specific test to eliminate any contra-indications before proceeding, and if there is the slightest risk another method will be selected. In the low back, rotary techniques may include the 'side posture' or 'lumbar roll' adjustment, which involves torquing the spine from shoulder to pelvis in such a way as to isolate the specific joint, whereupon pressure is directly applied over it, or the spinous ... thrust is accompanied by an ... it on by leaning against the

... nding name, the Break is an ... the facet joint on the opposite ... eck sideways. It eliminates the ... n some circumstances be ill-advised.

Telephone Malvern (0684) 567480

17, Alexandra Road,
Malvern,
Worcs. WR14 1HA

In Manu Vis Medendi

Dawn Akers
Oxford (01865) 245926 —

McTIMONEY TECHNIQUE
CHIROPRACTIC MANIPULATION

DIVERSIFIED TECHNIQUES

Scores of techniques use the same principles of taking the joint to its maximum stretch before applying a final rapid but shallow thrust, and these involve variable positional techniques, contact points, and lines of drive to bring about a specific predetermined move. Most require a hand to stabilize or apply leverage, whilst the Contact hand directs the force of the adjustment. These Diversified techniques, which include direct thrust techniques such as the Rotary and Break, form the basis of a chiropractor's training, and Alfred States's popular student manual describes 87 different moves on the spine and pelvis alone. For example, he describes 8 different moves to adjust the base of the skull on the first vertebra, 16 techniques to adjust the lumbar spine, and 18 to adjust the thorax, preparing the student with the bare essentials of a suitable technique for almost every eventuality.

DROP TECHNIQUE

The chiropractic profession has developed specialized equipment to refine some of its direct thrust techniques, particularly the Toggle Recoil. One example is the Drop Table, where sections corresponding to the neck, thorax, and lumbar spine may be sprung at a specific tension. The moment during the adjustment that tension is overcome, the section lying under the

Adjustment of the Talus bone in the ankle

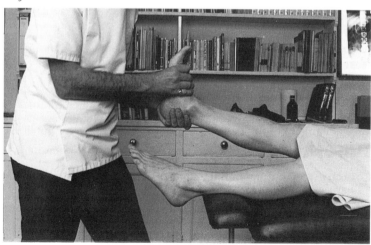

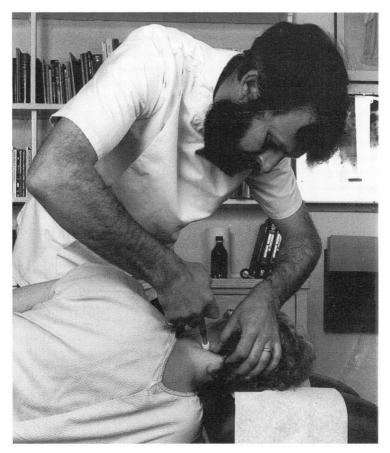

Using the Activator

part of the patient's spine being adjusted gives way and drops about an inch. This not only limits the force applied to a pre-set level, but it enhances the adjustment through the recoil that is induced. The Thompson Drop Table technique was one of the first treatment systems employing such a table, and remains its most popular example.

ACTIVATOR

One instrument that is particularly useful when manual adjustment is ill-advised is the Activator. Set to deliver a measured light thrust, it is held in the hand and applied directly to the joint. Cases of advanced osteoarthritis or thinning of the bone (osteoporosis) respond particularly well and painlessly where a manual method might prove uncomfortable or risky. Although its inventors have evolved a detailed system of analysis and treatment around it, many chiropractors use it only when the conventional approach is inappropriate, and a 1986 questionnaire by the 1,000 strong Ontario Chiropractic Association suggested that 25 per cent of their members made use of it in practice.

ADJUSTING INSTRUMENTS

Even more complex instruments have been designed to deliver a preset force in a specific direction and are built into a specially designed couch. Relying on intricate X-ray measurements of the neck and skull together with careful patient positioning, the results in previously unresponsive cases are often highly dramatic. Due to the specialized nature of these instruments they are not readily available, and in Britain only about 3 per cent of chiropractors have access to them. In America they are more widely used.

Instruments should always be regarded as useful refinements, and few chiropractors are shackled to any one technique. In 1974, the morning after chiropractor Dinos Ramon was forced to abandon his newly equipped clinic in the North of Cyprus, he was bringing relief to his fellow refugees on an earthen floor using nothing but his bare hands, in the way that his training had taught him. Prior to this Dr Ramon had preferred the use of specialized equipment, but forced to leave this behind him he was able to deliver a full and effective service with just his hands.

NIMMO RECEPTOR TONUS METHOD

The Receptor Tonus method of treatment devised by Raymond Nimmo is a soft tissue approach that uses stimulation of reflex points to free locked vertebrae, tighten slack ones, and clear subluxations. Specific nodules – or trigger points – are located either close to or far from the spine and a steady 5 second pressure using the weight of the relaxed arm is applied through a finger, thumb, or instrument. This initiates a response through the autonomic nervous system to restore normal neurological activity. Some have likened these trigger points to fuses in an electrical circuit, which are 'blown' and eliminated by the high electrical stimulus of the manual pressure applied to them. With the removal of the irritant trigger point, normal neurological activity is restored to the associated vertebral unit, which then functions fully again.

SACRO-OCCIPITAL TECHNIQUE

Within the field of chiropractic numerous post-graduate techniques of analysis and treatment have come and gone. One which has survived is the Sacro-Occipital Technique of Dr Major Dejarnette. It is designed to diagnose and treat disorders associated with the impeded flow of cerebro-spinal fluid, and involves adjusting both directly and indirectly cranial, sacral, and spinal mechanisms. Fulfilling the desire of those who do not wish to restrict their practices to musculo-skeletal conditions alone, SOT seminars are becoming very well attended post-graduate study courses in many countries. Much of SOT's inspiration has come from the Cranial Osteopathy of Sutherland and others and, like Applied Kinesiology, it claims to have advanced the frontiers of cranial techniques.

APPLIED KINESIOLOGY

Perhaps the most successful of the post-graduate study techniques is Applied Kinesiology evolved by Dr George Goodheart. A chiropractor who delved deeply into Eastern and Western systems of alternative medicine, Goodheart integrated his studies into a highly complex system of analysis and treatment. Using a form of muscle testing, his methods, like those of Dejarnette, aim to treat the whole body and not just the musculo-skeletal system, and they involve cranial, reflex, and nutritional mechanisms. In its simplest form Applied Kinesiology muscle testing methods are the basis for 'Touch For Health', a short lay-persons' course now gaining popularity outside the chiropractic profession and used often as an indicator in allergy testing. However, the fully integrated Applied Kinesiology course embraces lengthy seminars for professionals, and is tied to a curriculum laid down by the International College of Applied Kinesiology which sets examination standards and issues post-graduate diplomas.

ADVICE ON STRESS AND LIFESTYLE

The chiropractor is trained to look at the root cause of a problem, and if a condition cannot be related to a specific incident, he or she will often make enquiries into working habits, ergonomics, diet, posture, stress and other environmental factors. It is sometimes very difficult to determine one specific cause, and there may be quite a number of trivial factors which combine to bring on the problem. One of the commonest is persistent stress, which heightens the body's fight and flight response. The postural muscles of the back are held in a state of sprung tension, with shoulders raised, neck extended, and buttocks tightened for the duration of the stress, and if there are any existing weaknesses in the spine inducing localized muscle reactions these will be multiplied many times over by such superimposed postural stresses. Quite minor problems that are rarely felt at all will, all of a sudden, become painfully evident and although adjustment or soft-tissue techniques may remove the symptoms, continued stress may well bring them on again.

Stress may not necessarily be restricted to psychological factors and may well relate to poor work surfaces, over-weight, ill-designed car seating, or the wrong type of vigorous exercise. Henri Gillet suspected that certain thoracic subluxations were linked to brands of margarine or coffee that irritated the digestive system as a form of low grade but potent stress. Other better known irritants are smoking, junk foods, and alcohol, and more and more people are found to be reacting to food additives, pollutants, modern building materials, synthetic fabrics, and the chemical spin-offs of technological advancement. When acting as stressors in a susceptible individual these irritants overload the system and can either exaggerate minor structural weaknesses or create subluxations in their own right. Although chiropractic adjustment will often bring relief, the problem may well recur until the root cause is found and corrected.

CONTRA-INDICATIONS

B.J. Palmer wrote in 1934: 'It is more important to know when not to adjust than when to adjust.' As with almost any valid method of treatment there are times when the conventional chiropractic approach may be ill-advised. For example, it is unwise for any manipulative procedure to be applied to a joint suffering active rheumatoid arthritis or acute ankylosing spondylitis. However, when the inflammation has subsided, certain chiropractic techniques can be most beneficial in rheumatoid arthritis, and the application of cryotherapy (cold packs) may even help during the active phase. Likewise, many sufferers of ankylosing spondylitis are able to lead relatively pain-free lives when regular careful treatment is applied. Advanced spondylitis, or arthritis, precludes the use of some of the more vigorous methods, but a chiropractor has so many soft-tissue, non-force, or gentle adjustment methods that the quality of life of a sufferer can still be dramatically improved. It is tragic that so many patients with 'arthritis', 'old age', or 'wear and tear' are told by their medical doctor to go home and learn to live with it, when correctly applied techniques by a qualified chiropractor can often make them feel like teenagers again. The same applies to sufferers of osteoporosis (thinning of the bones), for the appropriate chiropractic approach will normally bring about a dramatic reduction of pain with no risk to the patient.

Chiropractors, with their training in pathology, diagnosis, and radiographic interpretation, are ideally placed to detect the various cancers that may appear as muscle or joint pain. In practice, chiropractors regularly find that they are the first to discover a tumour when this has been overlooked by a patient's medical physician or specialist, and they are then able to direct the patient along the appropriate channels. Even when a cancer is found to be malignant chiropractic can sometimes be applied, not to cure the condition, but to reduce any discomfort whilst the patient is also undergoing conventional medical therapy. In these circumstances it is usually minimum force or indirect techniques that are applied near the diseased area rather than any vigorous methods.

Other forms of bone weakness such as metabolic demineralization, inflammatory bone diseases, tuberculosis of the bone, and fractures, rule out direct or forceful adjustment. Similarly, where the ligaments and tissues of a joint have been recently torn by a whiplash accident or other injury, and inflammation persists, these methods are to be avoided. There are certain circulatory disorders such as aneurism, advanced arteriosclerosis, or anticoagulant therapy where a safe and gentle approach must be chosen with great care.

Although many forms of dizziness and vertigo respond well to conventional chiropractic treatment, there are a small number that rule out rotary or forceful manoeuvres when treating the neck. In all cases of vertigo or dizziness the qualified chiropractor will first perform tests to rule these out, and if they prove positive will select techniques that present no threat.

Much has been made by medical opponents of the risks of stroke. They cite examples of stroke following rotary manipulation of the neck and use these to condemn the whole profession whilst neglecting to set their own house in order. An analysis of reported incidents indicates that in the 30 years from 1948 to 1978 there have been 25 cases world-wide following manipulation, seven by chiropractors and 18 by medical practitioners (of whom ten claimed to use chiropractic techniques). In view of medical hostility to chiropractic and medicine's ability to hush up its own mistakes the real figures are probably weighted even more heavily against medical manipulators. When taking into consideration the many, many, millions of neck manipulations that must have been performed around the world by chiropractors, the seven cases of stroke laid at their door represent an infinitesimal ratio, especially when it is appreciated that the 18 medical cases come from a profession which performs relatively little manipulation, and that during this 30 year period there were another seven cases of stroke brought on by sudden neck movement from the patient himself. Putting it in perspective, the renowned French orthopaedic physician Robert Maigne recorded: 'There is probably less than one death of this nature out of several tens of millions of manipulations.' David Chapman-Smith, an international lawyer specializing in chiropractic issues, stated: 'You have about as much chance of dying from chiropractic cervical adjustment as from a bee sting, or being hit by lightning. You have more chance of dying from the effort of giving the adjustment than your patient from receiving it.' Nevertheless, wary even of this very remote possibility, qualified chiropractors are trained to perform specific screening tests so that no inappropriate manipulation should ever be applied to susceptible patients. Neck manipulation by a properly qualified chiropractor is therefore quite safe, and in borderline cases non-force methods are selected that carry no risk whatever.

There are certain spinal abnormalities that chiropractors are particularly well qualified to recognize by their radiologic training. One very common finding is lack of symmetrical shape in the lower lumbar facet joints, and such patients often react painfully when the common side-lying lumbar roll is applied. When such findings appear on X-ray the patient may be adjusted by using a non-twisting method lying face down, face up, on the side, or sitting. Certain types of acute lumbar disc protrusion should never be adjusted in rotational side posture and another position will be chosen. In those cases which are accompanied by a cauda equina syndrome, with its symptoms of bowel or bladder loss of control, the chiropractor will waste no time in referring the patient for the appropriate surgical intervention.

A study in England by Dr Alan Breen of 600 consecutive patients revealed that 6 per cent had been referred to the National Health Service for conventional treatment. Twelve were cases of intractible disc prolapse, eight were cancers (prostate carcinoma, other bone secondaries, spinal cord tumour, and Ewings Sarcoma), six were advanced hip arthritis, four were Polymyalgia Rheumatica, and there were two cases each of advanced spondylolisthesis, fracture of the femoral neck and Multiple Sclerosis, and one case each of Osteomyelitis, Rheumatoid Arthritis, Ankylosing Spondylitis, Paget's Disease, Dural Block, and Aortic Aneurism. All had been previously undiagnosed, and although one quarter had previously been examined by their medical practitioner the diagnosis had either been missed or the condition had not been far enough advanced at the time of examination. When one considers that a condition such as Polymyalgia Rheumatica can induce retinal destruction and blindness if not medically treated, and that four cases appeared in this sample of 600 patients, the importance of a sound conventional diagnostic training for practitioners of complementary and alternative medicine is underlined.

REACTIONS TO TREATMENT

It is quite normal for a 'reaction' to occur after a successful adjustment, particularly in the early stages of treatment. Swiss chiropractic researchers Sandoz and Lorenz describe these as mild muscular aches and pains coming on shortly after treatment and lasting on average two to three days. However, the reaction can last from half a day to over a week, and it is brought about by stretching of the ligaments, muscles, and joint capsule of the hitherto locked joint. Sandoz and Lorenz make the point that such a reaction is usually a very good sign, adding that it often occurs in patients who go on to experience a good response to treatment.

Other common reactions to adjustment include a hot flush of perspiration coming on immediately in response to the effects on the autonomic nervous system. An outbreak of intestinal wind and sometimes diarrhoea may follow adjustment of the lower thoracic or lumbar regions and, in women, neck and upper back adjustment can induce an early or heavy period the day after treatment. Within a day of treatment there may occasionally be a short bout of abdominal discomfort, and on rarer occasions nausea or sickness. In those patients who suffer from a volatile autonomic nervous system there may be fainting, cold sweats, nausea, and heart palpitations, but such reactions are very rare and harmless, and are normally followed by the correction of other health problems related to autonomic disturbances. In other rare instances adjustment of the neck or upper back may induce an immediate cold chill and tremor lasting several minutes, which will naturally concern the patient but which is quite harmless. These reactions may accompany any form of manual therapy, whether by chiropractor, osteopath, physiotherapist, or medical manipulator, and demonstrate the intricate relationship of the autonomic nervous system to spinal structures. They serve as a further illustration of how disorders of the spine may act through that system to create symptoms of disease in any organ of the body.

Provided the adjustment is applied by a qualified and competent chiropractor there should be no real adverse reactions. However, inappropriate or repetitive adjustment to an already mobile joint may bring about its destabilization, and the substitution of skill by force can cause permanent damage.

MEDICAL MANIPULATION

Many medical doctors or physiotherapists across the world, recognizing the value of manipulation, have followed weekend courses in this speciality. Although in some cases they provide a useful first-aid relief to their patients, it is horrifying that they learn a few quite forceful, and often crude, techniques without first developing the examination and manipulative skills of a four- or five-year full-time chiropractic course. Indeed, such is the problem that one highly respected medical orthopaedic specialist, Dr John Mennell, has stated that learning manipulation 'is a formidable undertaking for an active medical practitioner', adding that 'anything but the use of correct technique places the patient in jeopardy'. In spite of this Dr M.F. Grayson stated in the *British Medical Journal*: 'Courses including manipulation (lasting about a week) are run for doctors and physiotherapists by the Cyriax Foundation and by the Society of Orthopaedic Medicine, and intensive weekend courses for doctors are held by the British Association of Manipulative Medicine.' Although from this time doctors will be manipulating patients, Dr Grayson goes on to admit: 'Doctors will then need six to nine months of regular practice to begin to feel that they are treating the right patients and doing so appropriately – and years to become fully experienced and confident.' One might well wonder at whose expense this is achieved!

In Australia, with its government funding for five-year undergraduate programmes in chiropractic and osteopathy, one might expect a different attitude, especially since one of the principal findings of neighbouring New Zealand's Commission of Inquiry into Chiropractic was that: 'Part time or vacation courses in spinal manual therapy for MDs, physiotherapists and other health professionals should not be encouraged.' Thus, when the *Australian Family Physician* developed a correspondence course for medical practitioners in 1985 the Australian Medical Association distanced itself from it. In spite of this the *Australian Family Physician* is now, five years later, advertising its three-day course, 'Back Pain and Spinal Manipulation for Doctors', endorsed by the Royal College of General Practitioners. Commenting on this advertisement, New Zealand attorney David Chapman-Smith stated: 'Let's be quite clear – many patients will suffer injury and pain from crude manipulation from practitioners attending such a course.'

Fortunately, qualified chiropractors follow an extensive four- or five-year full-time course that ensures that they learn not only how to manipulate, but when and why. It is only when they have developed a full proficiency under close guidance that they embark upon their college internship, treating real patients under supervision. Medical orthopaedic specialists with a lifetime's experience in manipulative therapy recognize this as the only way. Dr James Cyriax of England stated: 'To learn when to manipulate and when not, and what sort of manoeuvres to use, is a diagnostic problem involving years of study.' The Frenchman

Dr Robert Maigne declared that: 'Prolonged training under guidance is indispensable.' Canadian Dr John Bourdillon asserted: 'The accurate appreciation of joint stiffness and, even more, that of excess tension in the muscles requires training and . . . even with constant practice this training takes a long time.' In the next chapter we shall learn about chiropractic training and understand why the New Zealand Government Commission into Chiropractic concluded of the chiropractor that:

> No other health professional is as well qualified by his general training to carry out a diagnosis for spinal mechanical dysfunction or to perform spinal manual therapy.

Chapter 10

EDUCATING THE CHIROPRACTOR

Learning is like a great house that requires a great charge to keep it in constant repair. *Samuel Butler (1612–1680)*

Standards of chiropractic education world-wide are now parallel to those of medicine, dentistry, and other established allied professions. In the United States credits from at least two years of a Bachelor's degree course are needed before students are enrolled into a chiropractic college, and elsewhere, in Australia, Canada, England, and France, university or medical school entrance standards are required. The four- or five-year full-time training programme is geared to producing the highest quality chiropractor – one with a firm foundation in the established broad spectrum of chiropractic techniques, yet fully versed in medical 'basic sciences' and diagnostic studies. This person is a superb chiropractor, who has been equipped to recognize when a patient should be referred back into the medical system of health care. Wherever it has attained a formal status, the reputation of chiropractic education has become synonymous with that accorded to the other established professions.

There was a time, as with all the other professions, when public perception was less generous. In Charles Sale's popular book *The Specialist*, champion privy-builder Lem Putt is made to ponder in one of his bluer moods: 'maybe I should have took up chiropractry or veternary'. In 1930, when this classic companion to the smallest room was written, chiropractic was suffering an all-time low. Beaten down by a collapsed economy, a divided profession, the prospect of jail, and sinister *agents provocateurs*, American chiropractic colleges were collapsing all over the continent.

From a high of 3,100 students in 1922, even the great Palmer

School had to stare closure in the face when the student roll dropped below 300 in 1929. It was only B.J. Palmer's success in real estate dealing and the profits from his popular WOC (World of Chiropractic) radio station which allowed him to secure such a massive loss-making venture.

In retrospect the depressed economy was not the disaster to chiropractic it may have seemed at the time. Those colleges that survived were fitter, leaner, and more dedicated than ever before, and were to provide a strong post-war springboard from which chiropractic education could start its meteoric rise to present levels.

When D.D. Palmer established Dr Palmer's School and Cure in 1896 with a handful of students, few other than Palmer himself – that great dreamer – could have foreseen almost a century later more than 50,000 chiropractors the world over claiming descent from those humble beginnings on the fourth floor of the Putnam Building. Many of Palmer's earliest students were already medically qualified, and several, such as Alvah Gregory, Arthur Forster, A.P. Davis, and Alfred Walton, went on to plant chiropractic deep in the soil of basic medical science. The earliest chiropractic schools taught anatomy, physiology, and pathology, and some clearly outshone their medical rivals. In his survey of medical schools Abraham Flexner drew attention to the appallingly low quality of some medical schools, particularly in areas like Chicago, which Flexner called 'the plague spot to medical education in the country'. In spite of this, Chicago became the seat of the National School of Chiropractic which went on to excel in its teaching of the basic sciences, becoming the first chiropractic college to set the four-year full-time training standard in 1934. Many of chiropractic's earliest textbooks were written by medical physicians trained in chiropractic under D.D. or B.J. Palmer, and these became the first stepping stones on chiropractic's climb to educational fulfilment.

The first school to set itself up in competition to the Fountain-head was William Solon Langworthy's American School of Chiropractic and Nature Cure in Cedar Rapids, Iowa. Langworthy introduced a number of concepts into his teaching of chiropractic including the use of traction, and this attracted the displeasure of the Palmers. Through his journal *The Backbone* Langworthy was able to influence a number of early pioneers with his ideas.

Charles Ray Parker started the Parker School in Ottumwa, Iowa, only a few months after graduating from the Palmer School in 1905. It survived for three years during which it trained Willard Carver, and in the year of his graduation Carver was to be found providing legal advice to D.D. Palmer following his trial and imprisonment.

Not all of the early chiropractic schools were as conscientiously committed as these and a few were run primarily for profit. Some sacrificed genuine learning for quick financial returns and were little more than diploma mills. There is always this risk when a profession such as chiropractic remains unregistered, but as more and more chiropractic laws entered statute books across the American continent, so fewer fast bucks were made, and the less reputable courses collapsed with the onset of the Great Depression.

COUNCIL ON CHIROPRACTIC EDUCATION (CCE)

The earliest attempts to arrive at a common core curriculum which could be verified externally and subjected to quality control began in the late 1920s when the National Chiropractors' Association formed its Committee on Educational Standards under the able chairmanship of Dr John J. Nugent. It was unfortunate that during these years the Palmer School abandoned established chiropractic techniques in favour of B.J.'s Upper Cervical Specific Technique, and the School naturally became highly suspicious of any accreditation programme. Opposition arose through the Chiropractic Health Bureau, later the International Chiropractors Association, which represented the interests of those chiropractors influenced by the Palmer School.

John Nugent was vigorously attacked from all sides. His insistence that small colleges should merge, educational foundations become non profit-making, teaching become professionally based, standards be raised, and training be extended to a full four years was opposed by many a mixer school as well. His was once described 'the most hated name in chiropractic', yet his tireless efforts in the face of constant criticism were to bear fruit in the 1950s, when the full-time four-year course became standard throughout chiropractic education, and colleges throughout the United States began to pull themselves up by their bootstraps. An unsung hero during his lifetime, John Nugent's contribution has been one of the most significant in chiropractic history.

Hampered by the Second World War, all attempts to form an accrediting body ceased until 1947, when the establishment of the Council on Chiropractic Education laid the foundation for modern chiropractic training along the lines laid down by Nugent. Its standards were adopted by most of the colleges whose graduates formed the National Chiropractors' Association (NCA), but not by those supported by the International Chiropractors Association (ICA).

When the NCA was wound up in the early 1960s, most of its members went on to form the American Chiropractic Association and were joined by a significant number from the ICA. The newly formed association remained the largest professional body, with about three times the membership of its rival, and it was highly active in supporting and funding the Council on Chiropractic Education (CCE). By the end of the decade memories of B.J. Palmer were beginning to fade, and although Palmer College still did not seek CCE accreditation the Council was finally endorsed by the International Chiropractic Association. This set the stage for CCE's detachment from both political bodies, and they granted it autonomy in 1971.

As a totally independent body the Council on Chiropractic Education was ready to apply for formal recognition by the United States Office of Education. It achieved this status in 1974, whereupon the Palmer College saw the advantages of accreditation and formally applied. When this was granted in July 1979 the process of educational standardization started nearly fifty years before was at an end. It is a standardization which chiropractic the world over now acknowledges as necessary for the training of a safe, competent, broadly-based chiropractor, and it provides the educational foundation upon which are built the independent Canadian, Australasian, and European Councils on Chiropractic Education.

GOVERNMENT COMMISSIONS

In February 1987 the Swedish Government's Commission on Alternative Medicine reported:

As regards formal qualifications, it has been ascertained that Doctors of Chiropractic follow a four to five year course of university level training, which is regarded internationally as being of good quality. This training has already a couple of times also been examined by Swedish authorities and, in its preclinical parts, it has been found to be equivalent to the Swedish medical training.

The Commission concluded: 'The training and clinical work of Doctors of Chiropractic is of such a qualified nature that there are grounds for official recognition.' Furthermore, the Commission states: 'It is considered that chiropractors who have been registered will have such competence in differential diagnosis that they can work independently with their own medical professional responsibility.' They recommended that: 'Chiropractors who become registered should also be incorporated into the health insurance system in Sweden.' Sweden has no chiropractic college of its own, and the members of the Swedish Chiropractic Association are trained at the Anglo-European College of Chiropractic in England, in North America, or in Australia.

The most thorough examination ever conducted into chiropractic was that published in 1979 by the New Zealand Government's Commission of Inquiry. As with Sweden, New Zealand has no chiropractic college of its own, and the Commission needed to travel to Australia's International College, England's Anglo-European College, the Canadian Memorial College, and three United States colleges before concluding its findings on chiropractic education. Among their summary of principal findings are the following statements:

Modern chiropractic is far from being an 'unscientific cult'.

Chiropractors are the only health practitioners who are necessarily equipped by their education and training to carry out spinal manual therapy.

The education and training of a registered chiropractor are sufficient to enable him to determine whether there are contra-indications to spinal manual therapy in a particular case, and whether the patient should have medical care instead of or as well as chiropractic care.

The responsibility for spinal manual therapy training, because of its specialised nature, should lie with the chiropractic profession.

Part-time or vacation courses in spinal manual therapy for other health professionals should not be encouraged.

Both the Swedish and New Zealand studies were commissioned by government. The former included on its panel an orthopaedic surgeon, a neurologist, a physiotherapist, and a member of Sweden's Department of Health, yet in spite of this managed to retain independence from interference by the organized medical profession. The New Zealand study avoided the risk of any medical bias by appointing a lawyer, a scientist, and an educationist, and evidence was given under oath and subject to cross-examination. The three commissioners noted early on: 'As we prepared ourselves for this inquiry it became very clear that the forces of organized medicine were vigorously opposed to chiropractic.' Ever since chiropractic emerged as a distinct and independent approach it has had to deal with the forces of half-truth and misinformation, and in particular with the accusation that chiropractic is an unscientific quasi-religious cult. This could not be further from the truth today, but it is still being promulgated by certain sections of the American medical establishment.

SCIENTIFIC BASIS

Commenting upon the common scientific base of chiropractic and medicine the New Zealand Commission states:

> While the specifically chiropractic material is of course not taught outside chiropractic colleges there is much other material that is. Indeed, considerably more than half the contact hours in the 4 to 5 year course offered are concerned with just those topics which are to be found in any standard preclinical medical course. The chiropractic student is therefore well exposed to anatomy, physiology, pathology, microbiology, human biochemistry, and diagnosis (including laboratory procedures) and in a CCE college he will probably be taught these subjects by a non chiropractor using standard medical texts. He is therefore exposed to the whole range of scientifically based factual material that medical students are.

Chiropractic educationists firmly believe that if their graduates are to treat members of the public without medical referral, then they should leave college with enough knowledge to ensure that the interests and safety of the public are thoroughly preserved.

DIAGNOSIS

On the subject of diagnosis chiropractors the world over suffer from their exclusion from the hospital rounds. They are therefore introduced to advanced pathological conditions through textbooks, slides and video-recordings, but not often to the real-life situation. However, a point accepted by the New Zealand Commission was that hospital cases were totally different entities from those presenting themselves at a chiropractor's consulting rooms, for in hospital they have reached a stage that can only be managed at that level. Even though not of the hospital mould, the many patients that pass through the hands of chiropractic interns during their training prepare them admirably for a real-life situation, and it is towards these patients that a student's diagnostic training is directed. A medical student very often has to wait to enter general practice before receiving adequate exposure to everyday problems, and the New Zealand Commission agreed that: 'The chiropractor's training fits him as well and possibly better than does a medical training for diagnosis at the general practitioner level.' The commissioners added:

> If the chiropractor has been adequately trained to identify conditions which are beyond his powers to treat – and we believe he does receive such training at CCE colleges – then he is actually at an advantage over his medical opposite number when it comes to conditions which are biomechanical in origin. He is trained to treat such cases, whereas the medical practitioner – except in a few cases – is trained only to administer drugs for pain reflief.

EDUCATION IN THE UNITED STATES

Statistics published by the Foundation for the Advancement of Chiropractic Tenets and Science (FACTS) reveal that in Spring 1989, of the 10,914 chiropractic students enrolled world-wide, nearly 88 per cent were undertaking training at one of the 17 United States colleges. Fourteen of these colleges were fully accredited by the CCE, while three colleges, with only a total student enrolment of 461, limited themselves to what they term Straight chiropractic. By refusing to adopt standards of diagnostic training laid down by the Council on Chiropractic Education, the Straight colleges have restricted their graduates to practice within those few states with broader licensing laws. Indeed more and more of their graduates are now taking up the option of travel overseas to countries where chiropractic is not restricted to CCE level requirements, as they discover that they are unable to practise in their own home states. Unfortunately they bring their problems with them and often create differences of emphasis and standards of practice that disrupt the unity of the profession in their adopted countries.

In point of sheer size Palmer College of Chiropractic in Davenport, Iowa (founded 1897), and Life Chiropractic College, Marietta, Georgia (1974), with 1546 and 1357 students respectively, were clearly the leaders, with the Los Angeles College of Chiropractic, Glendale, California (1911), taking third place with 996 students. National College in Lombard, Illinois (1906), Logan College, Chesterfield, Missouri (1935), New York Chiropractic College, Glen Head, New York (1919), and North Western College, Bloomington, Minnesota (1941) lay in a band from 707 to 543 students each, while Cleveland College split itself between Kansas City, Missouri (1922) and Los Angeles, California (1908), with 276 at the one and 354 students at the other location. Both Palmer and Life Colleges have Californian branches, Palmer West at Palo Alto (1978) with 518 and Life West at San Lorenzo (1973) with 428 students.

The remaining CCE accredited colleges, like their larger colleagues, are well-known names the world over. They include Parker College, Irving, Texas (1982), Western States College, Portland, Oregon (1903), and Texas College, Pasadena, Texas (1908), and their campuses range from 402 to 329 students.

Southern California College, Pasadena, California (1973), Sherman College, Spartanburg, South Carolina (1973) and Pennsylvania School, Leavittown, Pennsylvania (1978), with 165, 114, and 76 students represent less than 4 per cent of the total chiropractic student population in the United States. They have moved away from mainstream chiropractic education by rejecting the standards laid down by CCE, and as outcasts they initiated an accrediting agency, the Straight Chiropractic Academic Standards Association (SCASA). Amidst great controversy this body was granted a provisional two-year recognized status by retiring Secretary of Education William J. Bennett on 30 August 1988, against the recommendation of the Department's National Advisory Committee on Accreditation and Institutional Eligibility. It remains to be seen whether this recognition will help graduates from SCASA accredited colleges in their attempts to practise in the 30 or so states that currently deny them a licence, and whether the promised two-year status will be extended.

Within the United States every state has its own licensing laws for chiropractors, which require licencees to pass the state examination. The standards of these examinations range widely, some states requiring a very deep knowledge of the basic medical sciences, whilst others are content with a more scanty level of understanding. The wide divergence is a residue of the division left by the Straights and Mixers controversy, now perpetuated by the SCASA/CCE differences. Those state legislatures captured by the Straights tended to enact laws requiring minimal depth of diagnostic training.

Most states require graduation from a CCE accredited college, a pass in the examinations given by the National Board of Chiropractic Examiners, or both. The National Board examinations take the form of multiple choice questions, and are divided into two parts. The first concentrates on papers in General Anatomy, Spinal Anatomy, Physiology, Chemistry, Pathology, Microbiology, and Public Health, and is usually taken when the students are in their second year of study at a chiropractic college. The second part is normally taken during a student's final year at college, with examination papers in General Diagnosis, Neuromusculoskeletal Diagnosis, X-Ray, Chiropractic Principles, Chiropractic Practice, and Associated Clinical Sciences. In addition, there is an elective paper on Physiotherapy. The National Board examinations are taken at centres across the United States, as well as in England and Australia.

EDUCATION IN CANADA

With the formal federal endorsement of the United States Council on Chiropractic Education, Canadian chiropractors recognized the need to lay down their own standards to avoid becoming the repository for graduates from non-accredited colleges in the United States. The Council on Chiropractic Education (Canada) Inc. was formed to closely reflect its North American neighbour, and has become Canada's recognized accrediting agency. When CCE Canada and US-CCE formally agreed reciprocal recognition in June 1982, another milestone had been reached.

The Canadian Memorial Chiropractic College (CMCC), established in Toronto, Ontario in September 1945, at the end of the Second World War, is the only established college in the nation, and has been training chiropractors who have settled the world over. The Memorial title is a tribute to the fact that D.D. Palmer was Canadian born. With 588 students enrolled in Spring 1989, CMCC represents the largest chiropractic college outside the United States, and for many years it has emphasized its strong academic leaning, as 75 per cent of its undergraduates already have other degrees. It is one of eight recognized anatomy schools in the province of Ontario, having been accredited under Ontario's Anatomy Act in 1950, and it is thereby able to conduct human dissection for teaching purposes like its United States counterparts.

In addition to passing their internal college and individual Canadian state licensure examinations, most Canadian chiropractors are expected to sit the ten two-hour written examinations set by the Canadian Chiropractic Examining Board. All papers must be passed with a minimum 50 per cent score, and there must then be an overall average of 60 per cent to ensure success. To be eligible, candidates must be graduates of a CCE Canada accredited college, and the examinations are held at CMCC in Toronto, in Calgary Alberta, at Palmer College of Chiropractic, United States and at the Anglo-European College of Chiropractic, England.

The CMCC moved to its present custom-built premises in 1968, and 169 faculty and staff members were teaching around 600 students in 1989. When the college received full accreditation from CCE Canada in November 1986 its President, Dr Ian D. Coulter, hailed this as: 'The most important step in the history of CMCC . . . the last form of legitimization that we can get, other than university affiliation.'

The college was the first to recognize the need for a thorough database on chiropractic research, and in 1974 published its first biographical index. As the Chiropractic Research Abstracts Collection (CRAC), this index is regarded as the most authoritative index of chiropractic research world-wide.

A two-year postgraduate residency programme in either chiropractic sciences or radiography was established in 1974, and on completion successful residents sit for an examination that leads to certification as Fellow of the College of Chiropractic Sciences (Canada) or Fellow of the College of Chiropractic Radiology (Canada). The programme involves six months at the University Hospital, Saskatchewan.

During the 1970s the Ontario Council on Health and the Ontario Council of Universities expressed the need for chiropractic to be located with the province's established university structure. In spite of willingness by CMCC to explore this road to full integration, obstructions were placed in its way by the Ministry of Universities and Colleges. As a result there is a very real possibility that CMCC will move to the University of Victoria in British Columbia to realize its ambition.

EDUCATION IN EUROPE

In 1989 the third largest college outside the United States was the Anglo-European College of Chiropractic in Bournemouth, England. With a campus nearing 300, their students were drawn from 19 nations, and about half were British. The question of whether there should or should not be a European college dates back to the late 1920s, and since American training and textbooks were all in the English language the United Kingdom was an obvious choice. Here agreement ceased, for it was not until the death of B.J. Palmer that serious attempts were made to establish one.

European chiropractors, with few exceptions, were trained at Palmer School and tied their allegiance closely to B.J. Palmer. Clearly they considered that the best education available was to be received at the Fountainhead. Nevertheless, colleges purporting to teach chiropractic did emerge in the 1930s. The British Chiropractic College in London provided a training of 'twenty-five extension lessons in graduated lecture formation, profusely illustrated with many drawings and diagrams', for which the fee was £8. Also at this time the Edinburgh College of Naturopathy, Osteopathy and Chiropractic was awarding its

Triple Diplomate (ND,DO,DC) after a short course of study. However, a more serious institution did establish itself in 1925, and was graduating chiropractors the following year. The British College of Chiropractic was London based, and although its members had contemplated forming their own association, this was shelved when the Dean learned of the newly formed and Palmer-sponsored British Chiropractors' Association. There was polite correspondence between the two organizations, but the college was never recognized by the BCA and soon faded into oblivion during the economic collapse of the Depression.

An internal report was submitted to the officers of the British Chiropractors' Association on 2 July 1932, concluding that any school should be privately run, under British control, but with European representation proportional to each national association's investment in it. London was the preferred site, with Oxford or Birmingham as popular alternatives. Staffing would ideally be by a British faculty, but it was thought that few would be prepared to relinquish a lucrative practice. There were immigration problems in importing Americans, and a feeling that British chiropractors would lose face if unable to provide their own instructors. It was suggested that a floating capital of £20,000 would be needed, and that any short-fall could be made up by issuing shares to chiropractors from Britain or the European continent. It was recommended that the school curriculum:

> Should be run on straight chiropractic principles, teaching such subjects as are essential to graduate a highly trained practitioner, without the superfluous grinding into unnecessary subjects, but sufficient to give us a sound fighting argument to place before the Ministry of Health, if we are to seek legal recognition.

The report warned that chiropractors 'have to face the result of the national and world-wide depression', calling it 'a serious problem'. The committee advised caution, 'a careful scrutiny of all the facts', and 'a firm conviction that the needed co-operation will be forthcoming in all respects'. They and their colleagues had seen so many fly-by-night operations in the United States and Britain that they refused to rush ahead until all the conditions were right.

ANGLO-EUROPEAN COLLEGE OF CHIROPRACTIC

The conditions were never right, for although the profession expanded gradually to a pre-war peak its membership was halved to 34 by 1945. As early as 1917, when the British School of Osteopathy was founded by Martin Littlejohn, osteopathic colleges had begun to offer a British alternative to that long and financially draining trek to America. However the British chiropractic profession stagnated until the courage and determination of two chiropractors, Robert Beech and Donald Bennett, assured the establishment of the Anglo-European College of Chiropractic, and they registered it as a limited company in 1960. With many chiropractors firmly opposed to the concept, these two pioneers, supported by colleagues in Britain and Europe, raised funds from the profession and patients, and premises were purchased close to Robert Beech's Bournemouth practice. Doors were opened to its first class in September 1965, and the following year a neighbouring property was purchased, providing facilities for an out-patient clinic, X-ray unit, and laboratories.

The college gradually expanded until it was nearly bursting at the seams. Achieving high international academic successes it still lacked the attractive campus and student sporting and recreational facilities enjoyed by chiropractic students elsewhere in the world. An ambitious and daring covenanting scheme was devised by Plymouth chiropractor George Walker, and massive sums were pledged by a mere 90 British chiropractors. By topping up with donations from individuals in Europe and the Danish Pro-Chiropractic Association, a patient support group, a quarter of a million pounds was raised in 1981 to purchase and equip new premises nearby. Now with open spaces and superb facilities and under the determined leadership of Arne Christensen the AECC was ready to move towards recognition of its diploma as a Bachelor of Science degree. In May 1988 the Council for National Academic Awards accredited the course, making the AECC the first complementary or alternative medicine college in Europe to offer a validated degree. With its superb research facilities it is now moving towards the accreditation of an Honours degree, and its recent successes were underlined when HRH The Princess of Wales agreed to become its patron.

AECC students are assessed and examined throughout their four year full-time course. They begin their chiropractic studies immediately, developing techniques of palpation and muscle testing, but do not start working on adjusting skills until the beginning of the second year. This is to stress the point that, using visual and tactile perception, you must first learn why and when to adjust before you address yourself to how you deliver that adjustment. By the end of the students' second year they are encouraged to observe a senior Intern's out-patient treatments, and within six weeks of starting their third year they must have performed their first case history, examination, and written case report. They continue to develop their technical and diagnostic skills during this third year until, in the third term, they are presented for the clinic entrance examination. This vigorous practical examination involves the candidate moving from station to station whilst he performs a multitude of clinical tasks such as case history taking, physical examination, diagnosis, and reporting findings. Those who are successful proceed into the out-patient clinic as Junior Interns, treating, under skilled supervision, both new patients and those already undergoing treatment.

By the time students enter their fourth year they are ready, as Senior Interns, to manage patients in their own right, though still under supervision. The conditions under which they work are as close as possible to those they will meet in private practice, and they have at their fingertips all the modern diagnostic and treatment facilities they could possibly need. The AECC college clinic deals with over 30,000 out-patient visits each year drawn from the residents of the South Dorset-Hampshire area, and the experience gained produces a competent and confident graduate fully prepared for real practice. The average number of patient visits managed by any one under-graduate is thought to outstrip the figures of most chiropractic colleges in the world.

There are plans to introduce a fifth year in the near future at approved centres across Europe. This will be not unlike the British General Practitioner Training Scheme, whereby the new graduate will undergo a further twelve months of practical postgraduate tuition by an experienced and specially trained chiropractor at an established practice. It will also bear similarities to the rigorous post-graduate training that Swiss chiropractors must undergo, and which must be passed before a new graduate can be licensed to practise as a chiropractor in Switzerland.

One of the aims of the AECC is to qualify students with a thorough understanding of research methodology, so that they can go on to contribute to the research base of the profession. Much criticism has been levelled at chiropractic for failing to get to grips with serious research. Until now chiropractic has lacked the financial backing enjoyed by more established professions, but this is no excuse to ignore it. It has therefore been AECC's policy since inception to inculcate into students the thrill of research. This has been done largely by giving each student a major area of original research to explore during the final eighteen months, and this must be written up under the guidance of tutors as a thesis, to be presented and defended before an external examining board.

On the academic side the AECC has long been recognized for its quality graduates who regularly excel in the American and Canadian Board examinations. Basic medical sciences and medical diagnosis are taught by qualified specialists in those fields, allowing the chiropractic faculty to concentrate upon the science and art of chiropractic without distraction. Unlike any college teaching 'alternative' or 'complementary' medicine in Britain, the AECC faculty staff are full-time, with experienced chiropractors able to give of their best without the distraction of running a general practice. A research department, under the full-time guidance of chiropractor Alan Breen, ensures that the AECC is at the forefront of international chiropractic research. His epidemiological studies into chiropractic, published in a well-known scientific journal during the 1970s, and his involvement in the Medical Research Council's comparative trials in the 1980s have established his scientific reputation well beyond the chiropractic profession.

FRENCH INSTITUTE OF CHIROPRACTIC

The French Chiropractic Association initiated a year-long pre-college course in 1979 to prepare Baccalaureate level students for any of the established chiropractic colleges. This was expanded in December 1983 into a full-time five-year course by adding another four years based closely on the American CCE model. The French Institute, a private non-profit organization, graduated its first students in November 1987 and they received their diplomas after passing the external examination of the European Board of Chiropractic Examiners.

SCANDINAVIAN CHIROPRACTIC COLLEGE

Following the findings of Commissions of Inquiry in Norway and Sweden that recommended the establishment of local training facilities for chiropractors, and with the provision of National Health Service cover for chiropractic patients in Denmark well established, the Nordic Council, which co-ordinates the government policies of Denmark, Norway, Sweden, and Finland, considered the future of chiropractic education in Scandinavia. A unanimous resolution was made in March 1989 that a university faculty of chiropractic should be established.

Steps are now being taken to establish such a faculty at the University of Odense, one of three medical schools in Denmark. It already provides the one-year pre-chiropractic course required by the authorities for students planning to practise after their four-year chiropractic training, and it is now set to become the hub of chiropractic training for the whole of Scandinavia when it opens its doors in 1991 or 1992.

EUROPEAN BOARD OF CHIROPRACTIC EXAMINERS

The European Board of Examiners was established by the European Chiropractors' Union to ensure that graduates from European colleges have been trained to the high standards demanded by a profession in general practice. The examination takes the form of a lengthy interview by a panel of experienced examiners, enabling them to challenge the wide range of a student's knowledge and to probe for any weaknesses. Students are also expected to demonstrate their broad skills in the many chiropractic techniques taught, and they are brought before a second panel to defend their thesis. Once the Board is satisfied with a student's competence it will endorse the diploma, thereby enabling the graduate to join their national chiropractic association and to gain the respect of the international chiropractic community.

EUROPEAN COUNCIL ON CHIROPRACTIC EDUCATION

Europe has lagged behind in establishing a formal Council largely because the European Chiropractors' Union had laid down minimum educational standards for the members of its national chiropractic associations when it was formed in 1932. However, the need for an independent accrediting agency was recognized formally in 1981 at Avignon, and a subcommittee was formed to make recommendations. A provisional standard was approved in 1986 and its Board members appointed. CCE-Europe received full approval from all European chiropractic associations in 1988, and was formally established as an autonomous accrediting body and registered as such in Switzerland in 1989. Both the Anglo-European College and the French Institute have applied for the status of candidates for accreditation.

AUSTRALASIA

Chiropractic education in Australia has suffered from the emergence of home-trained chiropractors who have not followed the internationally recognized educational model. This has led to mixed levels of practice dependent upon the standards set by the individual states of Australia, and has created a confusion of identity between home-grown chiropractors and osteopaths who have largely come from the same mill.

In 1959 the Sydney College of Osteopathy, incorporating the Pan College, began teaching osteopathy and chiropractic as a privately-run establishment under the leadership of Alfred Kaufmann. However, in the following year a Royal Commission in Western Australia found that only chiropractors and dieticians possessed an education that suited them for registration, thereby raising the public's perception of chiropractic across the continent. Shortly after this the Sydney College changed its name to the Sydney College of Chiropractic and Osteopathy. Today it has abandoned its osteopathic title altogether, and is known as the Sydney College of Chiropractic, with a diploma accredited by the Higher Education Board of New South Wales. In Spring 1989 it was training 63 students, all of whom were required to have a BSc (Anatomy) degree or equivalent before embarking on the full-time two-year chiropractic curriculum.

At the same time as the Sydney College opened its doors the Chiropractic and Osteopathic College of Australasia established itself in Melbourne, and it too was to change its name, becoming the Chiropractic College of Australasia. Four years later another college entered the home-grown market as the Chiropractic, Osteopathic and Naturopathic College of South Australia, and this was to incorporate itself later as the Chiropractic and Osteopathic College of South Australia.

Amongst the background of this confusion the Australian Chiropractors' Association maintained its aloofness from non-representative chiropractic, and continued to adhere to internationally accepted standards of training and ethical discipline. The student trust fund established by the Chiropractors' Association of Victoria in 1954 helped to fund Australian students in America, and this was adopted by a number of other state associations to avoid complete swamping by those who were content to stay below mainstream chiropractic standards.

Patients from New South Wales began to mobilize against the plethora of dubious qualifications that were beginning to emerge, and in July 1970 formed a lay organization, the Committee for the Registration of Chiropractors (CROC) which grew to some 38,000 members. In November 1972 CROC awarded a personal certificate to each member of Parliament entitling them to practise chiropractic, thereby bringing home to the state's lawmakers the simplicity with which 'chiropractors' could be foisted upon the community. The following year the Premier appointed a Committee of Inquiry into the Question of the Registration of Chiropractors. When it published its findings in 1975 it recommended chiropractic registration and minimum standards of education. As the Sydney College of Chiropractic had trained the largest number of persons practising in influential and populous New South Wales it was recommended that theirs should be the minimum standard of education acceptable.

PHILLIP INSTITUTE OF TECHNOLOGY (VICTORIA)

The dogged persistence of the Australian Chiropractors' Association not to compromise its high standards eventually paid off. A massive fund-raising programme led to the establishment of an internationally acceptable five-year full-time chiropractic course run in conjunction with a university programme at the Preston (later Phillip) Institute of Technology in Melbourne, under the direction of Dr Andres Kleynhans.

In May 1979 the first graduates from the International Chiropractic College received diplomas that were of a high enough standard to ensure acceptance by mainstream chiropractic. Using the facilities of the Phillip Institute, the ICC at Bundoora received accreditation of their course by the Victoria Institute of Colleges, endowing their graduates with a recognized Bachelor of Applied Science (Chiropractic) degree. The college has subsequently been accredited both by the Australian Council on Tertiary Awards and by the Australasian Council on Chiropractic Education. When state funding was granted in 1980 the ICC changed its title to the School of Chiropractic and Osteopathy, and an osteopathic course was established to run alongside the chiropractic one.

AUSTRALASIAN COUNCIL ON CHIROPRACTIC EDUCATION

The Australian and New Zealand Chiropractors' Associations recognized the need to establish their own Council back in 1967, when the process was initiated. They formed the Australasian Committee on Chiropractic Education in 1972 to establish a course of international standard. By 1974 its job had been done, and the two associations decided the following year to establish an independent body of four chiropractors and four prominent lay people to monitor and advise on chiropractic education.

As the Australasian Council on Chiropractic Education, the Council liaised with government agencies, state registration boards, the chiropractic profession, and the public at large. One of its early roles was to report for the New Zealand Chiropractic Board on the educational programme at the ICC. Raising its membership to five professional and five lay persons it again inspected the ICC, now the School of Chiropractic,

205

and awarded it full accreditation in 1984.

In January 1986 the Australasian Council agreed reciprocal recognition with the Council on Chiropractic Education in the United States of America, putting the finishing touches to the triumphant battle of the Australian Chiropractors' Association against the state of mediocrity that had threatened to engulf Australia. Reciprocal recognition of the ACCE has indirectly enhanced the international status of the School of Chiropractic at the Phillip Institute, whose student roll in Spring 1989 stood at 304, making it the second largest chiropractic school outside the United States.

The only college to survive from the early years is the Sydney College. In 1989 it announced its intention to attach itself to Macquaire University, where the new Centre for Chiropractic Studies will operate the course. The first graduates of this programme will receive an M.Sc. Chiropractic degree and Sydney College is now seeking accreditation by the ACCE.

ASIAN CHIROPRACTIC TRAINING

Chiropractic has failed to develop as a separate entity in the Indian sub-continent, where traditional medicine incorporates aspects of manipulative therapy. This applies to South East Asia and China as well, although chiropractic has a foothold in Japan, probably because of post-war American influences. With a strong tradition of bonesetting firmly rooted in oriental culture, there is a plethora of institutions throughout Asia teaching a wide variety of methods. Many bonesetters are self-trained or have learned through an apprenticeship, and the only formal attempts to train chiropractors in Asia have been made in Japan. There are believed to be at least five chiropractic schools in the country. These vary so widely in course structure and content that a resolution of the 1984 Pacific Asian Regional Chiropractic Conference called for a review of the standards and status of the various institutions in the area, particularly in Japan where no standards have yet been laid down.

CHIROPRACTIC EDUCATION IN JAPAN

One Japanese course offers training in chiropractic adjustment techniques at a postgraduate level. Another follows a course structure embracing a mere 100 hours of training. One of the more advanced chiropractic courses in Japan is the full-time two-year course provided by the Japanese School of Chiropractic in Tokyo, which grants its own D.C. degree. The Chukyo Chiropractic College is also highly respected and has been training chiropractors for ten years, partly along lines laid down by the United States Council on Chiropractic Education. However, no Japanese course has yet achieved international status and the picture is further confused as manipulative techniques labelled 'chiropractic' are often taught in acupuncture, massage and pressure-point therapy courses, and there are correspondence courses of 'chiropractic and physical therapy' open to anyone willing to pay the tuition fee. This free-for-all situation in Japan has left the way wide open for technique-peddling mavericks to enter the market from America, selling short courses to all and sundry and issuing dubious and meaningless certificates.

TECHNIKON NATAL, SOUTH AFRICA

South Africa's Associated Health Service Professions Board invited all universities and Technikons in 1985 to consider introducing a chiropractic course. The following year the Board visited all respondents and selected the Technikon Natal as being most fitted for the purpose. After a massive fund-raising exercise, a five-year degree course leading to a Master's Diploma in Chiropractic was established at Technikon Natal, and the first 33 students enrolled in 1989. There will be reliance on private funding until government subsidies become available in 1994, when the first students qualify.

DOCTOR OF CHIROPRACTIC (D.C.) DEGREE

The D.C. degree awarded by accredited chiropractic colleges entitles the recipients to describe themselves as 'Doctor of

Chiropractic', and amongst themselves chiropractors the world over address each other as Doctor. The title is firmly rooted in the United States, where a doctoral degree is not necessarily a postgraduate research degree, but elsewhere opinions vary as to whether the title should or should not be publicly used. Taking the Latin root of the word to mean 'teacher' some have argued that use of the title should be restricted to those who teach. Others feel that as over 90 per cent of the world's chiropractors use the title as a matter of right all those with a common training should share that same right.

In Scandinavia the problem does not exist as a professional person claims their profession as their title, and would be introduced, for example, as 'Chiropractor Jensen'. In those parts of the world where the public perceive the word Doctor as applying only to medical practitioners the problem remains of confusing chiropractors with medical doctors. In Britain and several Commonwealth nations the majority of medical practitioners do not hold a doctorate in medicine, yet due to their accepted standards of training they adopt the title Doctor as one of courtesy. The issue is further complicated in Britain where the surgeons have proudly relinquished their doctor title to become Mister, even where they hold a formal M.D. (Doctor of Medicine) degree.

In those countries where confusion between Doctors of Medicine and Doctors of Chiropractic occurs, chiropractors are encouraged to qualify their title wherever possible by adding the words 'of Chiropractic', and the New Zealand Commission of Inquiry recommended that the title should be used with care. In Britain the profession is divided over use of the title, with one group stoutly defending the usage, whilst another sees itself as specialists eager to take on the 'Mister' title so proudly borne by British surgeons.

INTERNATIONAL TRENDS

Chiropractic education has been firmly established in the English language, and its standard texts are all published in English. Only one college has survived to teach chiropractic in another tongue, and that is the fledgeling French Institute, although their students are required to speak English and few texts are in French. Failure to develop the teaching of chiropractic in other tongues has serious stunted the growth of the profession, and there are large areas of the world where chiropractic is conspicuously absent. South and Central America have suffered as no Spanish-language college has ever survived long enough to establish training in Spanish.

Attempts began in 1927 with the foundation of the Daniel David Palmer Spanish-American School of Chiropractic in Mexico City, but it was financially unstable and folded six years later in 1933. Economic considerations remained a serious problem, and were recognized at the Pan American Regional Chiropractic Conference at Cancun in 1983 when local chiropractors reported that the massive devaluation of the Mexican peso against the US dollar was penalizing Mexicans training in the United States. However, a watershed was reached in 1988 when, not only did 17 chiropractors receive a licence to practise, but the Colegio De Profesionistas: Cientifico-Quiropracticos De Mexico, A.C. was formed as a Mexican CCE equivalent. This has paved the way for a new Mexican school, and if this is successful the door will at last be open to Latin Americans to spread chiropractic across the central and southern continent.

The Middle East and North Africa are also sparsely catered for by chiropractors, and the development of an Arabic language college would have excellent potential if it were to receive government support free of medical interference. Chiropractic has totally failed to take root in the Indian sub-continent, where traditional bonesetters fulfil the role. Africa is also largely undeveloped from a chiropractic point of view, although in South Africa chiropractic has recently been formally recognized by the government. Unfortunately, due to the political climate in Africa, other countries in that continent are unlikely to benefit from the South African College.

In Eastern Europe chiropractic principles and practice have been partially blended along with the medical model, although only on a limited scale. It is unlikely that any independent form of chiropractic education will ever develop in those countries, although chiropractic techniques will continue to enter orthopaedic training at some institutions.

The next twenty years are certain to see chiropractic taught in several languages across Europe and Scandinavia, where a number of governments will soon be registering the profession. During this time we shall probably witness the successful spread of chiropractic education into South America. Japan will probably strengthen its chiropractic education, but the rest of Asia is unlikely to contribute significantly to the chiropractic world.

Chapter 11

BUILDING THE PROFESSION

When bad men combine the good must associate; else they will fall, one by one, an unpitied sacrifice in a contemptible struggle.
Edmund Burke (1729–1797)

D.D. Palmer's vision for chiropractic was that it should sweep throughout the world, releasing mankind from the misery and despair of disease. The early profession quickly organized itself into a body it believed would be the vehicle for this dream, and 1906 saw the formation of the Universal Chiropractors' Association. Devoted to the practising and preaching of chiropractic in its purest form, without contamination from any modality either allopathic or eclectic, its members were highly critical of those who would even dare to hint that a medical or natural method might fall within the parameters of chiropractic treatment.

Many of D.D. Palmer's first students were medically trained, and he would even boast of medical praise on receiving credit from individual medical physicians. A number of these pupils went on to found or administer some of the first chiropractic schools that were beginning to spring up across the North American continent, and D.D. was to join one of these pupils in such a venture when evicted from his own Palmer School. Naturally their training and background influenced the type of graduate chiropractor who entered that early arena, a chiropractor prepared to enquire beyond blind faith into how and why the body worked, and capable of accepting non-chiropractic methods that alleviated suffering.

Another pioneer to go beyond the early remit of chiropractic was Willard Carver. When formulating chiropractic's own Trinity of Giants, early chiropractic historians have referred to Willard Carver as 'The Constructor'. His first profession as a successful lawyer gave him a broad enquiring mind, leading him to investigate a number of naturopathic approaches, including the importance of observing man's structural and postural make-up. These he incorporated into the teaching of chiropractic at his Oklahoma school as Carver's Scientific Catechism, and they became the focus of heated debate between himself and both Palmers, providing an excuse for the division of the profession into Straights and Mixers.

That excuse came with the growing influence of the Universal Chiropractors' Association, founded in 1906 to assist Straight chiropractors in their legal defence. Those with a medico-scientific or Carverian background felt alienated by its adversarial tactics, and they grouped together as a rival association. By 1911 the voice of the Mixers was being projected through the American Chiropractors' Association. The following year the UCA voted to admit Mixers, intensifying strife within the organization but restricting the growth of the ACA.

By the mid 1920s the full force of medical opposition had been turned against chiropractors, and with their need for survival paramount, the two organizations fraternized closely. This was unpalatable medicine for many a Straight chiropractor to swallow, and B.J. resigned in 1925. The following year a number joined him to form the Chiropractic Health Bureau, later renamed the International Chiropractors Association, evoking the dream of its first predecessor in looking beyond the shores of the United States. The ACA merged with the UCA to form the National Chiropractic Association in 1930, a title it sustained until the 1960s when it reverted to its old Mixer title of the American Chiropractic Association. During the 1970s hardened attitudes started to change, so much so that today's ICA allows its members to use adjunctive methods and the two associations co-operate on almost every important national issue. Indeed nowadays a chiropractor's association is more likely to indicate his college of origin, with Palmer and Life colleges feeding the ICA, and ACA being joined by graduates of the other colleges. A significant number belong to both of these major professional bodies.

With the acceptance of Mixing techniques by the ICA and the granting to Palmer College of CCE status there was no longer a voice for those determined to adhere to old Straight chiropractic principles. This led to the formation of the Association of Straight Chiropractors, and although it is numerically insignificant when compared to the membership of the other two national associations its mere existence serves to perpetuate damaging divisions within the profession. It is unlikely to grow to match the other bodies, as its members are derived in the main from the three small SCASA based colleges Sherman, Southern California and Pennsylvania.

CHIROPRACTIC IN BRITAIN

The first chiropractors to reach the shores of Britain were in the mould of the Universal Chiropractors' Association, having been trained by B.J. Palmer in Davenport. Martin Littlejohn's foresight and determination in founding the British School of Osteopathy in 1917 was already establishing the roots of osteopathy deep in British society, so that by 1925 the first of the Osteopathic Bills was being prepared for Parliament. Seeing this as a threat to their continued existence British chiropractors thereupon invited B.J. and Mabel Palmer to England to endorse their stand.

Preparations for the arrival of chiropractic's President and First Lady were conducted in the London rooms of J.H. Wilkinson, 250 Marylebone Road, and it was here that 19 founding members established the British Chiropractors' Association (now incorporated as the British Chiropractic Association). Its purpose was to 'handle Chiropractic, assist its growth, and be prepared for protective measures'. Arriving later in 1925 the Palmers gave their blessing to the new association, advising that it play a waiting game over the threatened Osteopaths Bill.

The Osteopaths Bill fell but the BCA survived, and with its Palmer pedigree it is not surprising that its first constitution should have firmly stated:

> The definition of Chiropractic shall be as given in the Universal Chiropractors Association Model Bill, viz:- 'Chiropractic is defined to be the science of palpating and adjusting the articulations of the human spinal column by hand only. This definition is inclusive and any and all other methods are hereby declared not to be Chiropractic.'

This stand was further endorsed by the provision that: 'No applicant shall be admitted as a member of the Association who does not practise straight chiropractic, and whose methods of dealing with patients are not strictly confined to the adjustment of the spine by the application of the bare hands.' Admission was restricted to 'those possessing a diploma from a Chiropractic College recognised by the Universal Chiropractors' Association, and having undergone a residential course of not less than two years'. In 1927 this requirement was increased to a three-year full-time course in line with Palmer's new ruling on chiropractic education.

Not surprisingly the early years of chiropractic in Britain were troubled by controversy. One chiropractor and his wife were refused permission to join the Association because she was also a trained chiropodist, and the Association feared she would use this as an adjunct alongside the practice of chiropractic. Another applicant practised colonic irrigation, and yet another gave dietary advice. When Ronald Rice in all honesty admitted that he 'might adjust a foot or two if it is indicated, and with complete explanation of its distinction from the chiropractic principle', he was forced to retract this in writing before admittance was granted.

In spite of its restrictions the Association grew. Every year its two-day conference presented 'work of a practical and technical nature', fostering debates on philosophy and demonstrating chiropractic techniques. The year 1930 had seen the founding of *The Progressive*, renamed the *British Chiropractors' Association Journal*, and this contained 'general articles of chiropractic interest'. The profession thrived so that by the onset of the Second World War the BCA boasted some 72 members, was financially robust, published an established chiropractic journal, and held regular conferences that were avidly attended. However, Hitler's Germany was not only to ravage the streets of London and Coventry, for his war was to decimate chiropractic's ranks with the call-up of Britons and the voluntary repatriation of overseas chiropractors.

The General Election of 1945 that swept away Winston Churchill also swept away chiropractic health insurance cover when it brought in a Labour Government and the Welfare State. In the previous 33 years of government regulated National Insurance Schemes, the Approved Health Insurance Societies had retained the right to pay benefit to subscribers wishing alternative treatment. Britain's new National Health Service relied upon a National Insurance Scheme which incorporated these insurance services. Under its terms Health Minister

Aneurin Bevan restricted a patient's freedom of choice to practitioners within the Service, thereby endorsing the medical establishment and excluding all those who were not registered medical practitioners. The worker was now obliged to make a compulsory state payment for Social Insurance that would not cover chiropractic treatment, yet could no longer secure chiropractic cover, for the old Health Insurance Society had ceased to exist. To make matters worse any worker claiming injury benefit was now committed to following 'any direction given him by the medical practitioner in attendance, and any prescribed rules of behaviour'. Claimants were 'to submit themselves from time to time to appropriate medical treatment for the said injury'.

The British Health Freedom Society was formed to fight the loss of patients' rights to benefit from non-medical treatment. They objected strongly to the loss of freedom of choice, and particularly to the penalties proposed for non-conformists, which 'include the loss of benefit, reduction of benefit and liability to a fine of up to five pounds per day for every day of disobedience to medical or bureaucratic institutions'.

The British Chiropractors' Association, with its aversion to any approach that was not strictly Straight chiropractic, had hitherto turned its back on all other medical or non-medical professions. With its numbers halved to 36, each facing hard times, circumstances now called for a radical rethink of isolationist policies. In December 1945 Miss A.N. Goddard and Miss Eileen Davis broke this solitary mould. On behalf of the BCA they joined the inaugural meeting of the Joint Committee of Unorthodox Practitioner Associations chaired by Labour Party Member of Parliament Mr George House. Miss Goddard was to write pointedly in her report: 'Chiropractic now figures in the list of the British Health Freedom Movement. Up till now it has been conspicuous by its absence.' Some days later she showed signs of exasperation, shared by many since those troubled times, when she wrote: 'Mr House will be a marvel if he manages to get some kind of unity into that heterogenous collection – the Unorthodox Practitioner!'

In spite of suffering the same fate as all those who have since embarked upon that stony road of unity in complementary and alternative medicine, Mr House and his Parliamentary colleague Mr F.C.R Douglas succeeded in overcoming the cruellest aspects of the proposed law. The provision that claimants were bound to follow medical directions was deleted. So was the criminal fine clause, which by now the medical lobby had raised, threatening every defaulter with 'a ten pound fine for every day's refusal to submit to the medical treatment considered good for him'. Now, in order to receive his benefit the claimant had to 'establish reasonable cause for refusing to follow prescribed treatment'. Had the unity Mr House called for been forthcoming it is quite possible that the outcome would have been more favourable.

Chiropractors and their bedfellows in the Health Freedom Movement received a few token concessions. The Ministry of Labour upheld their right to continue issuing incapacity certificates for benefit, a right which chiropractors still exercise today. However, treatment was no longer covered by those health insurance schemes which had been fully absorbed into the compulsory National Insurance System. This had clear repercussions for those whom the Welfare State had set out to protect. The British Health Freedom Society was to lament: 'Well-to-do people are not concerned over this problem . . . but workers cannot afford to pay both their insurance contributions and their unorthodox practitioners.' The Labour Party had won the 1945 election on its mandate of a Welfare State. To carry this out it needed concessions from the all-powerful medical profession. The Civil Service haggled as always to save face for the two contenders, but political reality dictates that those with the smallest voice are sacrificed. To this day in Britain chiropractic treatment is readily available to the financially well-off, but to the low-waged, unemployed, and needy it remains virtually unobtainable.

The National Health Service Act had two immediate repercussions for the chiropractic profession. On the one hand it was made considerably harder for a chiropractor to earn a living, and while the nation passed through the economic hardships of these post-War years the profession failed to thrive. On the other hand political expediency had dictated a need to turn for allegiance to other threatened professions. This now created a climate where chiropractic Mixing ceased to be looked upon as such a heinous crime. The hold of Straight chiropractic gradually waned so that as a new influx of chiropractors accompanied national economic improvement the old controversies were buried. By the time the Anglo-European College of Chiropractic opened its doors in 1965 a wide variety of approaches was possible, although then as now chiropractic adjustment remains the single most important aspect of treatment.

As the chiropractic profession entered the 1970s it began to grow, fed by new graduates trained at AECC. It had found attitudes softening amongst general medical practitioners, although their trade union the British Medical Association insisted on maintaining the full medical monopoly. In spite of this a ruling in 1977 by the governing body of medicine, the General Medical Council, enabled registered medical practitioners to refer patients to a chiropractor provided they are satisfied that the chiropractor is an appropriate person to deal with the patient's complaint and that the medical practitioner retains ultimate responsibility. The way was now clear for medical practitioners to refer patients officially to chiropractors without incurring disciplinary action.

This softening by medicine has also been accompanied by a softening of chiropractic attitudes. In 1974, after a strongly argued case by its president Stanley Lord, the British Chiropractors' Association decided by a majority vote of one to apply for registration to the Council formed under the 1960 Professions Supplementary to Medicine Act. Had the application been upheld and the conditions for chiropractic independence met, chiropractic would today be a registered profession, and as such ready to take the next step towards inclusion within the National Health Service. This was not to be, for the PSM Council rejected the application, refusing totally to give any reasons in spite of repeated requests to do so.

State registration is seen by the British Chiropractic Association as a means of stabilizing standards of ethics and training along internationally accepted lines. Not only will it enable discipline to be enforced, where hitherto offenders have merely resigned and then continued their unethical practices, but it protects the public from dangerous or misleading practitioners. Under Britain's Common Law anyone can call themselves a chiropractor, and as chiropractic has become better known its imitators have prospered. One part-time course recently described how its 'course is divided into two distinct schools, the bacaluareate (sic) level of seven months of part-time postal study by postal tuition which awards a BSc in chiropractic by examination. This is essentially a THEORETICAL instruction with the hands movements shewn either by sketches or photographs . . . to a person of average intelligence it is sufficient to commence and sustain practice'. Chiropractors have no wish to deprive such people from earning a living, for certain patients may be helped, but what they do wish to prevent is the inevitable instances of patient injury being laid at the door of the chiropractic profession. Such accusations continue to occur while accepted standards of chiropractic training and practice are ignored.

In its golden jubilee year of 1986 the General Council and Register of Osteopaths sponsored a Ten Minute Bill through Mr Roy Galley M.P. to register the osteopathic profession, and this was supported by the BCA. Lack of time prevented a second reading of the Bill, but the two professions in Britain are now working together towards government and parliamentary support of a Chiropractors and Osteopaths Bill which would establish independent Boards for the statutory registration of chiropractors and osteopaths in the United Kingdom. As might be expected, bodies within the alternative medicine movement whose standards fall short of those being called for have vociferously opposed these attempts at registration.

In Britain the profession has not been alone in seeking to achieve state registration. In the 1970s it was vigorously supported by the Chiropractic Advancement Association (then the British Pro-Chiropractic Association) in its attempts to obtain registration under the existing Professions Supplementary to Medicine legislation. Formed in 1965 by grateful chiropractic patients, the CAA boasts an impressive list of respected patrons and its membership is open to any member of the public wishing to advance the cause of chiropractic, providing they are not practising chiropractors. Several thousand members strong, the Association gives financial support to chiropractic research projects and to the Anglo-European College of Chiropractic. It is a member of the European Federation of Pro-Chiropractic Associations, which co-ordinates the several national patient support groups that play an active role in representing the needs of patients to the European Economic Community and other European bodies.

THE EUROPEAN CHIROPRACTORS' UNION

European chiropractors were invited by the British Chiropractors' Association to their annual conference in 1931 in order to lay the foundations for the European Chiropractors' Union. This was accomplished and the following year 21 chiropractors from Belgium, Denmark, Sweden, and Switzerland joined the sixth BCA conference for their inaugural meeting in the company of B.J. and Mabel Palmer. The Union has since grown beyond the founding five national associations to include Finland, France, West Germany, Greece, Holland, Ireland, Italy, Norway, and Spain, and the 14 nations follow a common policy through the ECU, setting educational standards, holding postgraduate conferences, funding chiropractic research, and supporting the attempts of each national member to achieve statutory registration. It represents over 1,200 chiropractors, with nearly half its members coming from Great Britain and Denmark. France, Norway, and Switzerland contribute more than a hundred members each, and Belgium, Holland, and Sweden more than fifty each. The profession is smaller in the remaining countries.

THE STRUGGLE IN SWITZERLAND

The first nation in Europe to provide state registration for chiropractors was Switzerland, but this was not without a long and bitter fight. The imprisonment of Simon Mueller in Mulen jail, Zurich, in 1933 not only made him the first European martyr for chiropractic, but stiffened the bond between European chiropractors. Mueller's letters graphically described his tiny dark 2 × 3 metre cell where 'cobwebs and spiders are the only friends'. Toilet facilities encompassed an 'ill-smelling old bucket and a jar of water', and his meals were so foul that he complained 'hardly would I want to mistreat my God-given system with such food!' These letters were sent by the eight members of the Swiss Chiropractic Association across Europe for eventual consumption by patients who represented 'a population of from fifty to five hundred thousand possible tourists whose goodwill towards Switzerland is lost'. The British Chiropractors' Association wrote to official bodies, including the Association of Hotelmen in Lucerne threatening dire consequences to the tourist traffic, and patients were encouraged to write from all over Europe. Prizes totalling US$200 were put up by the Swiss Association for those chiropractors organizing the most patient protest letters.

Harassment with massive fines and jail sentences continued, but public opinion in Switzerland was eventually swayed. The canton of Zurich, home of Simon Mueller, was the first to move towards a chiropractic law in 1935, although it did not reach the referendum stage until 1939, when a 56 per cent vote secured a positive result. The canton of Lucerne had become the first to pass a chiropractic law two years earlier, and gradually every one of the 26 cantons followed suit, with the final acceptance of Bern in 1974. Bern had long held out against legislation until the Swiss Pro-Chiropractic Association, a 10,000 strong patient support group, organized a petition for the inclusion of chiropractic under the National Sickness Insurance Scheme. Two months before the Bern elections the petition bearing nearly half a million signatures was handed in, representing one in every three Swiss citizens. Not only did this lead to a Swiss federal law for chiropractic, but it also ensured full recovery of fees under both state and private insurance schemes.

Today the profession is governed by the Inter-Canton Chiropractic Commission, composed of five chiropractors and five medical practitioners. This board approves the overseas chiropractic colleges from which chiropractors must graduate if they are to practise, sets its own national examinations, and ensures the completion of a two-year further training programme within an approved practice before granting a licence.

The Swiss experience has demonstrated a healthy co-operation between chiropractic and medicine. The year 1964 saw the official classification of chiropractors as primary care physicians independent of medicine, so that they have the right to refer patients to hospitals and to treat them there if the patient so requests. As a result inter-professional co-operation between medical and chiropractic physicians is stronger in Switzerland than anywhere else in the world.

HALF A CENTURY OF CONFLICT IN DENMARK

Within Scandinavia chiropractic has shown the greatest propensity for growth in Denmark. This has been made possible largely by the close co-operation that exists between the Danish Chiropractic Association and the patient support group, the

Danish Pro-Chiropractic Association. Both organizations were formed in 1925, largely in response to medical opposition in the form of salacious misinformation and the persecution of medical allies. One rumour was spread throughout a major hospital of a patient's blinding by a chiropractor who had prescribed a daily eyewash in urine. Another story was publicly circulated that a large consignment of canes had been delivered to a chiropractic clinic in Copenhagen, where patients were stripped naked before the chiropractor beat them until their blood ran. As a result of this campaign chiropractic clinics became known derogatorily as 'flogging clinics'.

In 1924 medical practitioner Dr J.M.B. Schilder was expelled from the Danish Medical Association for unethical behaviour in practising chiropractic, for there was 'no anatomical, physiological or experimental proof that chiropractic theories are anything but fancy'. The Court of Arbitration went on to state: 'Apart from the question of the validity of chiropractic theories, the examination of patients in the downtown clinics is in reality pointless, it has no significant purpose at all.' The *Danish Medical Journal* went on to publish the findings, stating that 'no medical practitioner practising chiropractic could be a member of the Danish Medical Association'. In spite of this chiropractors were able to overcome a strict Medical Act requiring all patients to have an initial medical examination through the courage and tenacity of Dr Schilder and three other medical physicians, Drs Faurby, Jacobsen, and Rames, who travelled to each chiropractic clinic in turn to pronounce waiting patients fit to receive chiropractic treatment.

Chiropractic continued to knock at the door of officialdom with a tiring regularity, backed by patient support from the Pro-Chiropractic Association. Time and time again the Ministry of Health refused to move, finding opportunities to stem the tide of pressure with delaying tactics, until they eventually passed the responsibility on to a Parliamentary Committee. As a result a new Medical Act came into force in 1935, and this enabled chiropractors to begin treating a patient without the need for a prior medical examination.

Meanwhile medical attacks continued. On the advice of the Health Care Directorate the heading 'Chiropractors' was removed from Copenhagen's classified telephone directory and the profession had to resort to law to achieve reinstatement. Attempts to broadcast on the radio were rejected, and countered by vicious attacks from medical doctors on the air-waves. One programme suggested that chiropractors kept a small stock of X-rays in circulation which were then shown to patients as their own. As always there was never any right of reply. One chiropractor was appointed secretary of his local Red Cross Society, a job which he ably fulfilled. However, a new attending physician was appointed to the Society in 1935 and after objections from him met with arbitration by an outside physician the Society was compelled to exclude the chiropractor against its wishes.

The Pro-Chiropractic Association continued to struggle through the 1940s, in 1941 securing 103,965 signatures in five months on a petition for the inclusion of chiropractic care under public health insurance. As reported in the Press, the Medical Association president responded by saying that: 'Those that feel better after chiropractic treatment will achieve exactly the same result by sticking their tongue out of the window for five minutes every day.'

As post-War currency restrictions effectively prevented students from embarking upon the long period of study in America, moral and financial support was given by the Pro-Chiropractic Association in 1948 for the foundation of the Dansk Kiroprakto Kursus (Danish Chiropractic College). The college served a useful purpose until conditions changed in 1951, and during its existence it graduated 15 chiropractors, each of whom had to achieve university entrance standards before being admitted onto the American-modelled course.

Inspired by the tireless efforts of chiropractic patient Vilhelm Krause, the Danish Pro-Chiropractic Association during the 1950s, 1960s, and 1970s continued to lobby officialdom. Submissions continued for the inclusion of chiropractic care within the Health Insurance Act, the more so after the publication of a long awaited Faculty Committee report in 1959. This report had been kept under close wraps since its completion in 1952, even though it had been commissioned in response to the chiropractic patient petition of 1941. As it relied heavily on a 1924 report and a Medical Council statement of 1930 it is not surprising that it strongly rejected any idea of formal recognition for chiropractic. It added that even if medical doctors referred a patient to a chiropractor, such a chiropractor still remained unqualified to practise. This report was so clearly out of date that the Government commissioned another the following year, and for the first time chiropractors were permitted to state their case. The new report was published in 1970 and recommended cover only upon medical referral, forcing the Danish Chiropractic Association to disassociate itself from the exercise. The Government had already put the recommended measures into effect the previous year, and the Association was able to show that in a four month period only 0.5 per cent of new patients had been medically referred.

The chiropractic and patient associations continued their struggle through the 1970s. By 1974 a new law was passed that provided a subsidy for X-ray examinations and up to four treatments in any year, but only if a chiropractic report was sent to the medical practitioner. Chiropractors were only prepared to accept this provision if medical doctors would send a report to the chiropractor. Agreement was not forthcoming and the recommendations were found to be unworkable. After further patient pressure an amendment was passed by Parliament in 1978, when the report requirement was deleted and the annual subsidized treatments raised to five. Since that date members of the Danish Chiropractic Association have worked independently of the medical profession and have enjoyed state subsidies, concluding the first stage of a battle which has raged for over half a century. The second stage has still to be won – that of state registration for the profession itself.

CHIROPRACTIC IN SCANDINAVIA

Norway became the first Scandinavian country to grant state registration to chiropractors when its parliament passed the Chiropractic Registration Act in 1988. This process had been set in motion by the Endresen Committee which proposed in 1984 that chiropractors should be free to refer patients to hospital for X-rays, CT scans, and other procedures. After much wrangling Norwegian chiropractors were removed from inclusion under the 'Quackery' laws and given protection of title early in 1988. State remuneration of fees applies only under medical referral. In view of the Danish experience the Norwegians have been given a year's trial, and if medical referral is not forthcoming it is likely that this provision will be deleted.

Sweden's parliament voted in 1989 for a Chiropractic Registration Act that took effect on 1 July that year, following the recommendation of its Commission on Alternative Medicine in 1987. This Commission, which included a strong medical and physiotherapy element, praised the quality of chiropractic education as being similar to medical training in Sweden. It recognized that the diagnostic competence of chiropractors qualified it for independence from medical referral, and recommended that chiropractic should not only be state registered but that patients should benefit from its inclusion under Sweden's health insurance system. The medical establishment has clearly learned from its experiences in Denmark where its opposition has been exposed as protectionist, and it has in this instance permitted educated men and women to reach their conclusions without interference.

The Finnish Chiropractic Association has only very recently been accepted into the European Chiropractors' Union as it had to wait for the requisite five members before becoming eligible for membership. Although relatively undeveloped in its provision of chiropractic care, Finland is likely to follow its Scandinavian neighbours with state registration. This will strengthen the profession, enabling it to grow and meet the nation's needs.

The recommendation by Scandinavia's Nordic Council, which co-ordinates the government policies of Denmark, Norway, Sweden, and Finland, that a programme of chiropractic training be set up within Scandinavia suggests a readiness for full acceptance of chiropractic within the four nation states. Once Scandinavia is able to train its own chiropractors the profession will be able to expand to cope with the needs of the public, and a standard internationally approved course will commence at Denmark's University of Odense.

CHIROPRACTIC ELSEWHERE IN EUROPE

With the exception of Switzerland, Sweden, Norway, and Liechtenstein, no European countries have a specific chiropractic law, and chiropractors either operate illegally or under forms of Common Law. In West Germany chiropractors are only permitted to practise if they first register under the 1939 Heilpraktiker (Health Practitioner) Law. There is no such law in

Belgium, where the Napoleonic Code operating there penalizes chiropractors, but since 1973 all 28 lawsuits have been successfully defended and an apparent tacit acceptance now exists.

Under the Roman-Dutch law of France any unregulated profession is illegal, and chiropractors have been fined up to 50,000 francs and have been jailed. Recently such penalties have usually been nominal and cases of legal harassment against individuals are less frequent. However, the profession of chiropractic is still exposed to less direct economic disadvantages by officialdom. One such example occurred in 1988 when the Minister of Health decreed that any mutual or health insurance company which reimbursed chiropractic treatment would be liable to penalties for aiding and abetting the practice of charlatanism. Chiropractic therefore remains out of the reach of the less-well-off French citizen.

In Greece the position remains uncertain. Charges were levelled by the Medical Association of Athens in 1987 against Dr Socrates Christodoularis, President of the Hellenic Chiropractic Association, and against another of the Association's seven members. When they were brought to trial in 1988 the Public Prosecutor appeared for the two defendants. After a fiercely contested hearing the charges were dropped. An appeal has been lodged which will lead to a decision by the High Court, and as recognition in Greece is determined by the judiciary rather than the legislature, the outcome of this case will be most significant for the future of chiropractic in Greece.

In Italy the practice of chiropractic is against the law unless it is sanctioned by medical referral. This has led to the emergence of medical clinics specializing in chiropractic, and many of Italy's 35 chiropractors work for organizations which bestow the mantle of medical protection upon them. Those chiropractors who choose to remain independent of such bodies make arrangements with favourable medical practitioners to their mutual benefit.

Elsewhere in Europe chiropractors are tolerated under forms of Common Law which permit the practice of any profession unless specifically prohibited. The Dutch were allowed to practise unhindered after the 1970 recommendation by the State Commission on Medical Practice that 'unqualified' persons should be prevented from practising only where the public are clearly at risk. Dutch chiropractors are awaiting the deliberations of a 1979 Committee on Alternative Health which is to make recommendations to Parliament. However, the situation continues whereby Dutch medical practitioners are practising unskilled manipulative therapy under the state sick fund scheme whilst trained chiropractic experts remain unqualified in the eyes of officialdom, as was acknowledged by Professor Jan van Es, the First Professor of General Practice in the Netherlands, at a London conference recently.

CHIROPRACTIC IN THE UNITED STATES

Chiropractic history in the United States is a catalogue of warfare between medicine and chiropractic over state legislation, punctuated by periods of civil war between the Straights and Mixers in the chiropractic camp. Each state is empowered to pass its own laws, but to do so for chiropractic they must first define precisely what chiropractic is.

The Straights were eager to tie chiropractic down to their own interpretation. In reporting to British chiropractors B.J. Palmer laid down the two principles generally accepted by American Supreme Courts when differentiating medicine from chiropractic:

> Cases constituting (1) Diagnosis, (2) The Treatment of Disease, (3) The Inhibition of Function, (4) The Stimulation of Function, and (5) The removal of portions of the body by operation, belong exclusively to physicians and surgeons. No other people have any prior right to any of these things.

Palmer defined the second principle, belonging exclusively to chiropractic:

> The discovery of the vertebral subluxation, that it impinges nerves, that it interferes with the flow of mental impulse affecting the quality of function at the periphery; the adjustment of the subluxation by hand only; the consequent enlargement of the foramen, the release of the mental impulse; restoration of normal impulse flow with restoration of the quality of function at the periphery, all constitute the PRIOR ART RIGHTS OF CHIROPRACTIC. These things are ours by right of discovery and development.

With such guiding principles before them, it was not surprising that those states adopting a Straight approach to chiropractic licensure entirely ruled out any concept of diagnosis and permitted no treatment other than the chiropractic adjustment.

On the other hand the Mixers were eager to broaden their definition of chiropractic to incorporate medical concepts, so that they could diagnose and treat named disorders and apply advice and treatment in addition to the chiropractic adjustment. Not only would they have to face the might of medical opposition to this, but also the Straights' powerful lobby. Often the hostility of the two chiropractic camps was so great that the medical profession needed to take little action to dissuade a state legislature from licensing chiropractic. In states with established chiropractic laws definitions of chiropractic are still to this day subject to redefinition or amendment, as one group succeeds for a while in gaining the upper hand on the other. This creates a situation where one day Mixers are freely prescribing vitamins, performing colonic irrigation, or delivering babies, yet the next day sees them prevented from practising anything other than straight chiropractic because the power of the Mixer lobby has been overcome by that of their chiropractic opponents. It can also create the anomaly of a respected institution such as New York Chiropractic College teaching the required CCE curriculum while New York's state laws deny chiropractors the right to practise parts of that CCE curriculum.

In spite of such internal difficulties, chiropractic licensing laws exist in all 50 states, as well as in the District of Columbia, the US Virgin Islands, and Puerto Rico. The first licensure application to come before a state legislature was that fostered by William Solon Langworthy in the state of Minnesota in 1906. It was killed off by the intervention of D.D. Palmer, who appealed in person to the state Governor to veto the Bill. Palmer could not bear the thought that the first chiropractic regulations should permit such a broad element of Mixing. The first successful state enactment was that of Kansas in 1913, but Arkansas was actually the first state to issue a chiropractic licence two years later. Connecticut, Florida, Idaho, Minnesota, Nebraska, North Dakota, Oklahoma, Oregon, Vermont, and Washington were soon to follow, and 39 states had some form of chiropractic legislation by 1931. It was not until 1974 that Louisiana completed the American story when it became the last state to register chiropractors.

Every state requires chiropractors to pass examinations set by its State Board. The nature of such boards varies, ranging from those with a total chiropractic component to others with a strong medical influence. In a few states a Basic Science Board examines all health professionals in the medical sciences, and may combine this with a separate board to examine the applicant in their own speciality, whether it be podiatry or chiropractic. Originally such boards were a move to exclude chiropractors from practice, but as chiropractic education advanced, so the Basic Sciences Board examinations became easier for chiropractors to pass. This led to the fall of such boards from a peak of 17 in 1950 to a mere 6 thirty years on.

The professional aspirations of chiropractors within each state are guided by local chiropractic associations, which tend to be formulated along traditional Straight/Mixer lines, and they meet as the Congress of Chiropractic State Associations. About 40 per cent of America's 45,000 chiropractors belonged to a national association in 1989. There are two major associations, the Mixers being represented by the larger American Chiropractic Association with an estimated 14,000 members (1989), whilst until the 1970s the interests of the Straights were pursued by the International Chiropractic Association with its strong Palmer College links. When Palmer College achieved full CCE accreditation in 1979 it turned its back on the strict Straight traditions. In the years since 1977 the chiropractic profession has doubled in size and it is not surprising that the CCE curriculum graduate has radically changed the emphasis of the ICA, so that both major associations allow their members to adopt either approach. The ICA is thought to be approximately 4,000 members strong (1989), and a number of chiropractors belong to both the major associations.

The process of rapprochement began in 1969 when ACA and ICA jointly produced the 'White Paper on the Health, Education, and Welfare Secretary's Report', challenging the accuracy of the United States Surgeon General's report of the previous year. From this time co-operation steadily increased, with the ICA taking up its seat on the ACA sponsored Council on Chiropractic Education, so that it was then possible to float the CCE as an independent external body in its own right in 1971. There were powerful moves to bring the two associations together under one broad grouping, and July 1987 saw a joint convention at Las Vegas where unity was thoroughly debated and many old wounds healed. A year later ICA members voted on merger with

ACA, and although 56 per cent of votes cast approved of this course there was insufficient support to achieve the required two-thirds majority for such a major decision. Although merger is unlikely in the immediate future, there is such a close co-operation between the two bodies over major national issues that there is a very real prospect of unity of purpose within the chiropractic profession before its centenary in 1995.

Although the two historic combatants have largely patched up their differences there still remains the problem of those strict Straights who have broken away from the ICA to form the Federation of Straight Chiropractic Organizations. Although only a tiny minority about 800 strong, this group is now being supplied by new blood from the three colleges accredited by the Straight Chiropractic Academic Standards Association (SCASA), perpetuating the old divisions. Much now depends on the ability of SCASA to make its provisional status from the Department of Education a permanent one, for if it fails it is quite likely that the Straight chiropractic cause will be lost for ever. Such an outcome would lay to rest a division within chiropractic which has beleaguered the profession from its earliest days, and would enhance its ability to defend itself against the encroachments of medicine and physiotherapy.

The territories occupied by chiropractors have been carved out by constant uphill battles against the American Medical Association, which has sought every opportunity to oppose state licensing, the broadening of state chiropractic definitions, the development of interprofessional co-operation, the entry of chiropractors into hospitals, and the reimbursement of fees. At a state level chiropractors have fought for health insurance equality, and inclusion under Workers Compensation schemes is now to be found in all 50 states. The majority of states, representing 70 per cent of the United States population, require that chiropractic services should be available under every commercial health and accident policy written in that state.

At a national level, chiropractors lobbied Congress to achieve federal reimbursement under Medicare, Medicaid, and vocational rehabilitation schemes. In 1985 Medicare, which provides health care for the aged, paid US$100 million in chiropractic reimbursements. Federal employees receive limited cover under Workers Compensation and Postmasters' and Mailhandlers' Benefit programmes, and major industrial companies provide chiropractic care for employees, as do many unions like the railroad and rubber unions. Veterans of the armed forces are entitled to chiropractic benefits, but only on medical referral from a doctor within the Veterans Administration programme, and veterans are entitled to grants to cover chiropractic education should they choose to become chiropractors on leaving the armed forces.

Chiropractic training for all other groups of people is not subsidized by government grant, unlike medical schools, although a 1984 law enabled chiropractic colleges to compete for funds to train students from disadvantaged backgrounds. Federal loans are available for chiropractic students, but these are high-interest only, unlike loans to medical students.

In the courts of law anti-trust suits have been filed against the medical establishment, seeking injunctions or damages against medical bodies for restraint of trade in their attempt to monopo-lize the health market in violation of federal anti-trust laws. The first, by five chiropractors led by Chester Wilk of Illinois, was filed in 1976 against the American Medical Association and twenty others, seeking an injunction against their illegal activities. At first it drew a Not Guilty verdict in 1981, but two years later this was overturned by Court of Appeal. Expensive litigation continued as the AMA and its co-defendants struggled to extricate themselves from court revelations of their conspiracy to eliminate chiropractic.

The case of the Chicago Five has uncovered organized medicine's own Watergate. With the full knowledge and backing of its executive officers, the AMA paid handsome salaries and expenses to a team whose express instructions were to destroy totally the chiropractic profession in America. The AMA formulated a Commission on Quackery in 1963 specifically to destroy chiropractic, as was evidenced by a memo from the head of AMA's Bureau of Investigation in 1971: 'Since the AMA Board of Trustees' decision . . . to establish a committee on quackery, your committee has considered its prime mission to be first the CONTAINMENT OF CHIROPRACTIC and ultimately the ELIMINATION OF CHIROPRACTIC (original emphasis).'

This and thousands of other incriminating documents found their way into chiropractic's hands, forming a clear picture of medicine's Mafia-like activities, and the massive extent of its crimes. Agents were sent around the nation to medical schools and professional organizations in order to specifically deride chiropractors with such terms as 'rabid dogs', 'killers', 'cultists', and 'unscientific quacks'. It is only human nature that medical practitioners at home and abroad should absorb this carefully concocted propaganda and that they should communicate it to media and patients alike. Some doctors became worried about their social contacts with chiropractors, and questions arose of the AMA such as: 'I am a member of the Rotary Club and a chiropractor has joined, must I resign?' The judicial council actually met to produce answers such as: 'You must resign only if the Rotary Club involves itself directly or indirectly in any health care matters, because then it would be a voluntary professional association with a cultist.'

Medical physicians were banned from teaching at chiropractic colleges, and those who were caught were black-listed and denied further employment in the medical system. The AMA admitted in one document that if they were to succeed they would need to prevent chiropractors from access to hospitals, and this they could enforce with their own punitive measures against recalcitrant hospital administrations.

Another goal was to keep chiropractors out of workers compensation, out of insurance policies, and out of state grants for their schools. 'We must stifle chiropractic education, we must keep them from attracting good students.' To sum up, this document ended with: 'Whatever you do, don't give professional recognition to chiropractors, never give them professional recognition.'

As these revelations unfolded, the AMA realized the extent of the damage done to them by their plots and machinations. Having offered nothing but the stick to the chiropractic donkey they were now forced to offer a carrot. In 1979 physicians were permitted to associate with chiropractors. However, this did nothing to undo decades of brainwashing inside and outside the medical profession. The president of the AMA in a magazine article even admitted that the new code of ethics had done nothing to change the attitude of doctors with regard to chiropractic. The AMA still continued to hamper attempts by chiropractors to have their credentials accepted by hospitals. As their court evidence was to demonstrate, they regarded chiropractic as a therapy akin to physiotherapy, and as such of no intrinsic value beyond what they, the medical profession, could themselves offer.

During the case it became clear that the AMA had done all in its power to stifle evidence of chiropractic's effectiveness. The

1966 report by AMA orthopaedic surgeon trustee Dr Hendryson, which said that injured servicemen during the war had responded impressively to chiropractic care, was buried. So was his observation on the effectiveness of chiropractic in eliminating pain and the need for bedrest in women suffering back pain during the later stages of pregnancy. Buried was the survey by the Kentucky Medical Association that showed 25 per cent of Kentucky's upper and middle clases regarded chiropractors as the specialists in treating muscle and joint pain. Evidence of cost-effectiveness from a senior orthopaedic surgeon, and actuary tables submitted to the Expert Review Panel by insurance companies were also overlooked. So was evidence that chiropractors were twice as effective as medicine and physiotherapy in returning injured workers to employment. As the case progressed it became clear that chiropractic care was far superior in this field, and that the AMA had knowingly put its interests as a trade association first, to the shameful detriment of the patients the Hippocratic Oath directs its members to serve.

In 1971 Dr Roland Martin, medical director of Oregon's Workers Compensation Board, concluded in a study that chiropractors were twice as efficient as medical physicians in returning to work people with comparable injuries. This was backed up by a massive study of workers compensation records in California published by Dr Wolf in 1975, again demonstrating that at every single study level chiropractors were twice as efficient.

The Illinois State Medical Society settled out of court in 1985, and several hospitals added doctors of chiropractic to their medical staffs. This now enabled patients at hospitals with access to chiropractors to be matched against comparable patients at hospitals without chiropractic care. Anatomy and orthopaedics expert Dr Per Freitag testified of his experiences at both types of hospital. He needed to give fewer epidural injections to pregnant women whose back pain had been treated by chiropractors in hospital, a fact he believed was important in the light of potential dangers to both mother and foetus from such injections. He testified that patients spent an average of five to seven days in John F. Kennedy Hospital, Chicago, where chiropractors were now on the staff, yet at nearby 'Lutheran General Hospital the same type of orthopedic patients spend an average of fourteen days' and do not have access to chiropractic care.

The full extent of medicine's illicit activity was emphasized in

1987 in Chicago. United States District Court Judge Susan Getzendanner ruled that the American Medical Association and its co-conspirators had violated the Sherman anti-trust laws of the United States by 'orchestrating a campaign to eliminate the chiropractic profession', causing an 'unreasonable restraint of trade'. She concluded that 'an injunction is necessary in this case. There are lingering effects of the conspiracy. The injury to the chiropractors' reputation has NOT been repaired.' The AMA was ordered to send their members a copy of the court's complete injunction, and to publish it in the *Journal of the American Medical Association*. They were also ordered to show to the Federal Court evidence that: 'It is now ethical for a medical physician to professionally associate with chiropractors, provided the physician believes it to be in the best interest of his patient.' Although the AMA have been obliged to fulfil these court orders they remain unrepentant and are continuing their fight in yet another costly appeal.

The Wilk case was the first anti-trust suit to reach the courts, but was not the only one. In 1979 the State Attorney of New York filed an action against 13 medical organizations and the Medical Society vice-president, seeking fines of up to US$13 million, and the state took this action 'as *parens patriae*, trustee, guardian, and representative of the welfare of its citizens'. Suits have been filed in several other states, and some have been settled out of court, enabling chiropractors to refer to hospitals, share laboratory and radiological facilities, and develop inter-professional relationships in many states.

Resort to the law has led to a scaling down of medical opposition in public, although it appears that dubious activities still continue behind the scenes and will probably not disappear until the generation tainted by misinformation has been succeeded by one accustomed to co-operating with chiropractors. Recently chiropractic investigator P.J. Lisa overcame police harassment to uncover documentation and build up taped evidence implicating the Indiana State Medical Society in an attempt to change unfavourably the legal definition of chiropractic. In his words: 'The Indiana State Medical Society hoped to rid themselves of an unwanted condition, chiropractic competition.' Yet in spite of these pockets of resistance, the legal climate and economic factors have brought about working relationships in hospitals, private medical establishments, and health organizations, giving patients a broad freedom of choice.

This is encouraged by the majority of insurance companies who now cover chiropractic, which they have found economically more effective in treating back conditions than standard medical care.

There are also signs that chiropractors may move into hospitals as a part of their training. At Lindell Hospital in St Louis, Missouri, doors were opened in 1983 when chiropractors were given admittance privileges, and 31 had affiliated to the hospital by 1984. Dr Russell Forbes, the hospital's chiropractic services department chief explained: 'Having gained access into the hospital, the next logical step was to see chiropractic residents working in the hospital on a day-to-day basis, 14 or 15 hours a day, seeing cases they would never see in their offices.' The first residency programme was launched in 1985 as a tough post-graduate training in family practice, and although Lindell is only one of 7,000 accredited hospitals in the USA, it has provided research opportunities, established interdisciplinary co-operation in a hospital setting, and allowed chiropractors to establish their worth as essential members of the health care team.

Similar programmes continued to develop through the 1980s. One of these followed a ruling in February 1989 by the Department of Health Services in the State of California, enabling chiropractors to join the medical faculty of the Pacific Hospital, Long Beach, California. Hospital administrator Gerald Goldberg has anticipated that many other hospitals will follow suit very quickly.

During the previous three years the hospital's radiology department had worked closely with chiropractors outside the hospital. Manager of the department Thomas King has stated:

> I'm very impressed with the equipment and training of the younger DCs. Their training is equal or better than that of young radiologists. The clinical indications usually match the pathology (found on the X-rays). Chiropractors are practising good radiology.

The Pacific Hospital exercise has also shown that it is possible for physiotherapists and chiropractors to work well in a hospital setting. Physiotherapist Linda Young, director of the department of physical medicine, was overjoyed by the degree of co-operation:

When I went to school it was DCs on one side and PTs on the other. Now it is whatever works for the patient. If a patient is treated by a PT, they may need to begin chiropractic treatment by a DC and vice versa. I sometimes appreciate chiropractors over MDs due to medicine's reliance on medication. I would rather get at the root cause.

As a result of this experience Mr Goldberg and the Chiropractic Section have established the first Hospital Chiropractic Education Programme. The chiropractic clinic at Pacific Hospital opened to students of Los Angeles College of Chiropractic in the summer of 1989, and the training programme includes undergraduate internship, undergraduate praeceptorship, and graduate praeceptorship. Mr Goldberg observed: 'The hospital is looked upon as a workshop for the medical profession. The key to the future is to bring chiropractic education into the hospital setting.'

CHIROPRACTIC IN CANADA

In Canada the profession organized itself into the Dominion Council of Canadian Chiropractors in January 1943. It received its federal charter ten years later as the Canadian Chiropractic Association. It is the only national association in Canada, and represents about 75 per cent of the profession. As with the United States each province enacts separate legislation, and chiropractors are licensed or registered in nine of the ten provinces. This started with Ontario in 1925, but Newfoundland with only twelve chiropractors has yet to complete the picture. Here the Newfoundland and Labrador Chiropractic Association is facing tough opposition in a province where the House Speaker, Finance Minister, and Health Minister are all medical doctors. In March 1987, one member of the House of Assembly stated: 'I think it is high time that this House took the bit between its teeth and used its undoubted powers to look into the possibility of this practice (chiropractic) being ended and these creatures being hounded out of our Province.' Naturally, while chiropractic remains unlicensed in Newfoundland, it remains vulnerable and patients are unable to benefit from provincial aid.

The four western provinces and Ontario contain two-thirds of Canada's population, and patients benefit from provincial medical aid programmes of fee reimbursement. However, there is no Government health cover in the less populated east of Canada, and although federal funds are made available for health and further education, only five provinces include cover for chiropractic. Nevertheless, there are 3,000 chiropractors at work in Canada, and chiropractic is readily available for most of the population, largely due to the success of the Canadian Memorial Chiropractic College.

To achieve licensure a Canadian chiropractor must have graduated from a college recognized by CCE (Canada) and must pass the examinations set by the Canadian Chiropractic Examining Board. In addition, most provinces require a pass in local oral or written examinations.

There is increasing co-operation between the chiropractic and medical professions in those provinces where chiropractic is established, and there are a small number of chiropractors working in university hospitals. The twelve-year research into chiropractic care for chronic back pain by Professor William Kirkaldy-Willis has done much to enhance the reputation of chiropractic since its publication in the mid 1980s.

CHIROPRACTIC IN CENTRAL AND SOUTH AMERICA

In Mexico chiropractic has received a mixed reception. Registration was initially provided for in 1955, but survived for one year only. It was then regranted in 1975, when chiropractors were registered with the Department of Professions and the Department of Sanitation, but in 1982 the register was closed for no reason. The 30 chiropractors registered at that time were still permitted to practise and take X-rays, but a quarter of the profession practised illegally as new arrivals until a third attempt at registration occurred early in 1988. At the end of November 1988 success was marked by the granting of licenses to 17 chiropractors, and by the establishment of a government endorsed CCE equivalent, the Colegio De Profesionistas: Cientifica-Quiropracticos De Mexico, A.C. Frequent medical referral in Mexico reflects the fact that there is little hostility towards chiropractors, and from 1982 there have been no prosecutions of illegal practitioners. Two bodies, the Scientific

Chiropractic Association of Mexico and the Chiropractic Association of Mexico, represent the interests of the profession, which now numbers about forty.

For a period of five years from 1927 Mexico City was the home of the Daniel David Palmer Spanish-American School of Chiropractic, but this, the only Spanish language college, was unable to weather the economic depression of the early 1930s. It is sad to reflect that had this college survived, the populations of Central and South America six decades later would possess the fully developed chiropractic health service desperately needed in that troubled continent. Signs are that this is soon to be remedied as there have been recent negotiations with a Mexican University to establish a chiropractic faculty.

In Central and South America there are few chiropractors. A planned chiropractic college in Brazil was foiled in 1964 when a military coup led to persecution and the departure of most chiropractors from Brazil.

The one chiropractor in Chile, Dr Victor H. Aguilera, has been constantly harassed by closure notices and fines which are doubled on every occasion. Initially granted a licence to practise in 1978, his success led to objections by the medical establishment, and his permit was withdrawn in 1981. He qualified and re-registered as a remedial masseur in order to continue serving his patients, but an arbitrary decision by the Central Health Service of Santiago forbade him to practise as of 2 April 1985. Nevertheless Dr Aguilera still fights on.

Although Colombia, Guatemala, Equador, and Venezuela do not regulate chiropractic, work permits allow foreign chiropractors to practise, and in Guatemala citizens may be given a limited permit through its 1967 Chiropractic Law. The Republic of Panama is the only Spanish speaking nation to fully license chiropractors, and this is dependent on passing the examination of the Panamanian Board of Chiropractic Examiners. The Chiropractic Association of Panama is the body representing local professional interests.

CHIROPRACTIC IN AUSTRALIA

It is believed that chiropractic entered Australia at the end of the First World War when Dr Harold Williams set up practice in Sydney. Although there are now 1,900 registered chiropractors, the profession remained small until 1961 when the Western Australia Royal Commission on Natural Therapy recommended chiropractic for registration. At that time there were about ninety qualified chiropractors spread throughout the continent.

The first national association was established in Sydney in 1938 by 22 chiropractors from New South Wales, Southern Australia, Victoria, and Western Australia, and membership was restricted to graduates of recognized American colleges. Its constitution strictly ruled that 'no applicant be admitted who does not practise what is known to the profession as Straight chiropractic'. This clause prompted the formation in 1943 of the Chiropractors' Association of Victoria when an application by a chiropractor named Hertzog was rejected in spite of strong lobbying by the Victoria members of the ACA.

Moves were initiated in 1959 by ACA president Stanley P. Bolton to bring the two camps together again. Shortly afterwards the 40 Victoria members joined the 53 ACA members under a revised constitution, clearing the way for the emergence of state branches of the ACA throughout Australia. The New South Wales and Victoria branches were founded in 1961 and 1962 respectively, followed by Western Australia and Southern Australia in 1964 and Queensland in 1966. The smaller states followed suit as the profession expanded, with branches in the Australian Capital Territories and in Tasmania forming in 1976, and with the Northern Territory completing the process in 1984.

During the late 1950s and early 1960s a number of schools of manipulation sprang up, creating a disparity of training standards within Australia. As the graduates of such schools were not trained to international standards they were barred from membership of the ACA, and the United Chiropractors' Association was formed in 1961 to represent them. Initially such chiropractors were fewer in number than Australian trained osteopaths, but the report by Western Australia's Royal Commission in favour of chiropractic led to a change of emphasis by naturopathic and osteopathic schools and many turned to training 'chiropractors'. Membership of the UCA now started to grow.

The first chiropractic state regulations followed the work of ACA founder Andrew Martin when, in 1945, chiropractors were exempted from the restrictions of the Western Australia Medical Act and were empowered to take X-rays. Legislation passed by the Parliament of South Australia in 1946 restricted manipulation to the physiotherapy profession, and existing chiropractors were only permitted to practise under a grandfather clause. Following representation by G.H. Thompson, South Australia passed the first Chiropractic Act on the Continent in 1949, although no regulatory machinery was laid down. A year later chiropractors were exempted from Western Australia's Physiotherapists Act, and the profession was defined within this legislation. New South Wales followed in 1956 when exemption from the NSW Medical Practitioners Act was granted to chiropractors, and the state defined chiropractic when exempting chiropractors from its 1959 Physiotherapists Act. This achievement was largely due to representations by ACA members John Fraser and Stanley W. Bolton. By the end of the 1950s various forms of statutory regulation had been granted to half of Australia's sovereign states, and all members of the ACA were empowered to take X-rays except those practising in Queensland and Tasmania. Tasmania's Health Minister denied a licence to X-ray patients to chiropractor Richard Le Breton in 1960, but this decision was overturned by the judiciary on appeal.

The first workable chiropractic registration act in Australia was passed by Western Australia in 1964, following the recommendation of its Royal Commission. However this state remained alone until 1978, when the Australian government Committee of Inquiry into Chiropractic, Osteopathy, Homoeopathy and Naturopathy chaired by Professor Edwin C. Webb published its findings, and legislation rapidly followed in the remaining states of Australia. Introduction in 1975 of the federal Medibank universal health insurance scheme prompted many insurers to include chiropractic benefit, and this process was completed by most other companies following Webb Report recommendations. State governments control Workers Compensation and Third Party accident insurance, and chiropractic treatment is available through these in most states.

Australia achieved the first wholly government-funded chiropractic education programme in the world with the School of Chiropractic and Osteopathy, known as the International College of Chiropractic until funding was granted in 1980. Established at Phillip Institute of Technology, its launch required considerable financial sacrifice from the Australian Chiropractors' Association. With 304 undergraduates enrolled on the chiropractic course in Spring 1989 this investment is now paying dividends by providing Australia with chiropractors of the highest possible calibre.

The Australian Chiropractors' Association with 900 members (1989), is strongly committed to maintaining internationally recognized standards of chiropractic training. The United Chiropractors' Association remains important, with 500 members. Both organizations have worked together on legislative and other matters for a number of years, but many ACA members are eager to preserve their chiropractic identity, and are opposed to the strong osteopathic influence prevailing in the UCA. More time will probably be needed before amalgamation of the two bodies becomes a realistic possibility, although wounds are healing.

CHIROPRACTIC IN NEW ZEALAND

New Zealand boasts a long chiropractic tradition, with the first practice being established in 1908 by Dr Otterhalt at Dunedin. The New Zealand Chiropractors' Association was incorporated in 1920. Forty years later the New Zealand Parliament passed the Chiropractors' Act registering the profession and creating a Chiropractic Board, but its administration was through the Department of Justice, since the Department of Health successfully opposed involvement. This unusual factor stunted the development of close inter-professional relations between medicine and chiropractic, but the position was remedied by the passage of a new Act in 1982. This followed Government Commission of Inquiry recommendations, and provided for a Chiropractic Board composed of four chiropractors, a lawyer, a medical practitioner, and an officer appointed by the Department of Health. Chiropractors must apply annually for a practice certificate to the Board, and an annual licence fee must also be obtained from the National Radiation Laboratory in order to take X-rays on the premises.

In 1975 the New Zealand Chiropractic Association obtained 95,000 signatures on a petition to include chiropractic in Social Security and Accident Compensation plans, and this led to the establishment in 1978 of a Government Commision of Inquiry into Chiropractic. Their findings were published in 1979, and represented the most thorough investigation into chiropractic ever undertaken. It stressed the safety, quality training, and specialist nature of chiropractic, and recommended that:

'Chiropractors should, in the public interest, be accepted as partners in the general health care system.' However, chiropractic fees are still only covered under the national Accident Compensation Corporation subject to medical referral, and this is a prerequisite for private insurance cover as well.

CHIROPRACTIC IN ASIA

In Asia there is a strong tradition of folk medicine which includes manipulation, and there is confusion as to what constitutes chiropractic. There are thousands of folk healers in Korea claiming to practise chiropractic, but none appear to have any training. A programme established by Life Chiropractic College at Taegu University in November 1986 aims to remedy the situation. This led to chiropractors joining the official South Korean Olympic team in September 1988, and 91 per cent of athletes receiving care at the Sang-Mu chiropractic clinic under the programme reported that chiropractic treatment improved their sporting performance.

In Japan, more than 2,000 practitioners advertise chiropractic, but only 50 hold any valid chiropractic qualifications. Here the Supreme Court has upheld a decision that any healing art is legal provided it does no harm, but qualified chiropractors have licensed themselves either as Oriental Medical Doctors, Acupuncturists, or Bonesetters. The Japanese Chiropractic Doctors' Association represents the officially trained profession, although there are at least five associations for others.

The Philippines also has a strong bonesetting tradition, and there are no legal requirements for chiropractic. Nevertheless there are only two qualified chiropractors in that country.

In Hong Kong qualified chiropractors have been in practice for more than fifty years, following the arrival of their first chiropractor, Dr Molthen, from the United States. There is an active Hong Kong Chiropractic Association which was formed in 1968 and now represents the Colony's 20 chiropractors. The Association has recently been pressing for legislation, but this has led to challenges in the courts over the right to practise chiropractic and the right to use the title *Ysang* (Doctor), as well as to police raids, interrogations, and arrests. Chiropractors are not entitled to take or interpret X-rays, although local radiographic laboratories often undertake this for them. There are attempts by the Association to formalize relations with the local medical community, but to date these have been rejected.

Two chiropractors opened the only clinic in Singapore in 1978, and are joined in their work from time to time by temporary associates from overseas. After attempting to establish the Singapore Chiropractic Association for eleven years, they finally achieved this in 1989, when the Singapore government formally sanctioned the Association.

Mainland China has no Western-style chiropractors, although within the Chinese Herb Physicians' Association there is a separate chiropractic division. Within the Association 'Internists' use chiropractic methods to treat organic conditions such as migraine and stomach cramps, and 'Surgeons' treat musculo-skeletal injuries with chiropractic adjustment. Life College established a programme at Beijing Institute of Traditional Chinese Medicine in 1988, and this is being run along the lines of its Korean curriculum.

In the rest of Asia and in the Indian sub-continent the practice of manipulation is widespread as a folk tradition, but chiropractic has failed to develop as a separate entity in spite of its position in much of the world as the most skilled expression of manual medicine.

CHIROPRACTIC IN AFRICA

Within Africa only Zimbabwe and South Africa have national chiropractic associations, and the profession is registered in both nations. Zimbabwe was the first to gain a free and open legislative status, unlike its South African neighbour. Chiropractic first arrived in the colony of Rhodesia in 1932 through Dr A. Scott, but no national association was formed until 1969. This spurred them into seeking an official status, and that was achieved by Act of Parliament six years later when the Chiropractic Council was set up to regulate the profession's affairs. This Council of five has two government nominees, while the remaining three are appointed by the Chiropractic Association of Zimbabwe. The Chiropractic Act allows the chiropractor to practise in the usual internationally accepted manner, and as such to take X-rays and use adjunctive physiotherapy. Reimbursement of chiropractic fees under state and private insurance funds is usual, including cover under army and air force medical aid plans. Prior to the independence of Zimbabwe in 1980 there were 17 chiropractors. In 1989 there were five.

South Africa attracted its first chiropractors shortly after the birth of the profession, yet it has had a chequered career there. The profession failed to expand in its early years, so that when medicine and dentistry were regulated in 1928 it was still too small to gain recognition. Within thirty years this position had changed, and chiropractors sought to formalize their status. In 1962 a Bill to register chiropractic was introduced to Parliament, but this prompted the establishment of a Commission of Inquiry. No chiropractic experts were consulted, no educational establishments were examined, and the process was conducted behind closed doors. It is therefore not surprising that South Africa produced the most medically-biased and ill-considered report ever conducted in the history of chiropractic. In 1971 renewed chiropractic pressure brought about a Chiropractors Act, but this was couched in such a way as to sound chiropractic's death knell. It provided a register for the 176 chiropractors, but then froze it so that no new chiropractors could be admitted, effectively strangling the profession. Having, as they thought, successfully eliminated the chiropractic profession the medical lobby then proceeded with the annihilation of other professions that threatened their monopoly. In 1982 the Associated Health Service Professions Board was established to control chiropractic, homoeopathy, naturopathy, osteopathy, and herbalism, again as 'terminal' legislation. The Board now fought back. It demanded a strong Code of Ethics, regulations for natural medicines, and a request for the Human Sciences Research Council of South Africa to conduct an inquiry on 'The experiences of South Africans relative to Chiropractic and Homoeopathy'.

In Parliament the medical establishment had successfully lobbied against the 'associated health professions' by playing on the 'charlatan' label. This was the label they had so cleverly pinned on chiropractic with that travesty of an inquiry twenty years before, but they were now to fall foul of it. Believing their own propaganda, the medical profession were delighted with the planned research project, seeing it as a final nail in the coffin of health competition. Yet the inquiry produced results that astonished them. One study involved the monitoring of patients who had tried orthodox medical treatment unsuccessfully on at least six occasions, and who then subsequently turned to chiropractic or homoeopathy. It was shown that chiropractic treatment had brought benefit to 88.76 per cent of medicine's failures, and with similar results for homoeopathy, medical opposition was exposed in its true light.

The chiropractic and homoeopathic registers were reopened by Act of Parliament in 1985. Training is to be provided at universities or technikons, starting with a six year course at Technikon Natal leading to a Master's Diploma in chiropractic. About 70 per cent of all medical insurances provide total or partial reimbursement of chiropractic fees. The South African chiropractic profession, reduced to 102 members by 1985, has now grown to 140 and is poised to expand into the twenty-first century.

The story is a different one in the rest of Africa, with the exception of Namibia where the law parallels that of South Africa. Five chiropractors were allowed to practise with few restrictions in Kenya, but recently prosecutions have been instigated after a policy change by the Ministry of Health, although foreign chiropractors have been left alone.

In Nigeria, one chiropractor has been permitted to establish a chiropractic department at one of the state hospitals, but a chiropractic review submitted to the Ministry of Health in 1983 has brought no official response; two other chiropractors practise outside the state system. Two chiropractors in Ethiopia were sponsored in 1957 by the Christian Chiropractors Association, and have remained in practice since in spite of remaining unregistered. Chiropractic cover in the rest of Africa is virtually non-existent.

CHIROPRACTIC IN THE MIDDLE EAST

Chiropractic has barely established itself in the Arab world, although in many nations, and particularly in Iraq, bonesetters are commonplace. The International Chiropractors Association started to remedy this by designing, staffing, and funding a preliminary trial of chiropractic treatment for low back pain at the Manchyatt Elbackray Hospital in Cairo in 1983. Impressed with the results Dr Medhad Alattar enrolled at Life Chiropractic College, becoming the first Egyptian to qualify in chiropractic, and several other Egyptian medical practitioners have followed his example by enrolling at Cleveland College. There are now plans to introduce chiropractors to government health clinics.

In the Gulf States a small number of chiropractors have been permitted to practise, having first obtained a local sponsor. Legislation now exists in the United Arab Emirates, and this permits chiropractors to treat neuro-musculo-skeletal disorders and to take X-rays.

In Jordan King Hussein has given his blessing to the registration of chiropractic, due to the respect and reputation of that nation's only chiropractor Dr Yussef Meshki. Protracted negotiations continued whilst the medical profession insisted on a medical referral clause, but finally agreement was reached in favour of chiropractic and in 1989 a suitable law was enacted.

Israel's 17 chiropractors remain unlicensed, although the Health Minister is currently forming guidelines. The previous government instituted an inquiry into chiropractic but, although completed, it remains unpublished. The Israel Chiropractic Association insists that legislation should secure chiropractors as independent primary health care providers, but a fear prevails that chiropractic may be made subject to medical referral. Currently manipulation is practised by physiotherapists in Israeli hospitals under medical referral, and there appears to be a very powerful anti-chiropractic medical lobby.

Many Iranian chiropractors left their country when the Shah was deposed, and only five remain. Although they are unregistered they are allowed to practise, and as there is a shortage of medical doctors they are accepted into the community and suffer no medical hostility. Chiropractic has yet to develop in Turkey.

Chiropractors have practised in Cyprus since Dinos Ramon returned to his native land in 1968. The Cyprus Chiropractic Association has sought registration, but a request in 1977 was turned down by the Ministry of Health as it was ruled that chiropractors were not practising medicine. The position was reversed by an amendment to the Medical Act in 1979, and now anyone diagnosing, treating, or giving medical advice is deemed to be practising medicine. This led to a second request in 1984, and the Minister ordered the Attorney General to create suitable chiropractic regulations. Meanwhile in 1985 Cyprus Chiropractic Association Secretary Phylaxis Ierides was charged with practising medicine without a licence, and then with taking X-rays without being medically licensed. In 1986 he was found guilty, but the judge declined to penalize him and recommended that chiropractic be registered. The Republic began to formulate a favourable chiropractic Bill, but shortly before its presentation to the House of Representatives a change in government brought a medical practitioner into office as Minister of Health. There was renewed insistence that chiropractic treatment be given only on medical referral, but it now seems that this may be dropped if Cypriot chiropractors abandon their right to take X-rays. The struggle continues for chiropractors to practise their profession without medical harassment, but sadly they may be forced to bend to the dictates of the medical profession by abandoning X-ray analysis on the premises, to the detriment of their patients.

EASTERN EUROPE AND USSR

In Eastern Europe there is no distinction between medicine and chiropractic, and some chiropractic concepts have been incorporated sporadically into health care provision. Influenced by the development of manual medicine in the two Germanies a strong manipulative faculty established itself in Czechoslovakia with Dr Karel Lewit the dominant figure. His teaching that spinal restriction is a source of irritation inducing autonomic nervous system responses is chiropractic in its purest form, and this concept is readily taken on board in countries where there is no health-care market, and therefore no financial threat from competition. However, in Yugoslavia a chiropractic health centre has been established at a Dubrovnik resort, and is licensed to treat tourists and Yugoslav citizens under arrangements with the Ministries of Health and Tourism. A number of Yugoslav students have been sent to America to study chiropractic so that the project can be expanded.

There are other isolated incidents of chiropractors working in Eastern Europe, one of the most recent being the contribution of Anisa Malahoff DC, an Australian of Russian descent, who offered her services following the Armenian earthquake disaster in 1988. Perhaps of greater significance was the welcome given to a delegation from the Federation Internationale de Chiropractic Sportive (FICS), when it arrived in Moscow in July 1989. Representing the international chiropractic profession in Olympic and other sporting events, FICS delegates were warmly received by the leaders of the two Soviet schools of manual medicine, and by representatives of a number of Soviet states and cities. During the awards banquet which followed, host Dr Anatoly Sitel announced his desire to 'commence negotiations to bring a DC programme to Moscow', possibly at Moscow University. It is hoped that further meetings between Soviet authorities, the European Chiropractors' Union, the World Federation of Chiropractic, and the United States Council on Chiropractic Education will lead to the establishment of a medically independent chiropractic college in the USSR that will integrate into the Soviet health care system.

FEDERATION INTERNATIONALE DE CHIROPRACTIC SPORTIVE

The federation, also known as the International Federation of Sports Chiropractic, was inaugurated at the International Chiropractic Conference in London in 1987 following energetic preparations by its President Dr Stephen Press. Its key aim is to provide first-class chiropractic health care for athletes worldwide by providing internationally recognized credentials that will be automatically accepted by all the international sports federations. So far more than forty national Olympic committees and many federal governments and international sports federations have accepted the FICS credential procedure.

During the 1988 Seoul Olympic Games 16 of its members were accredited to treat athletes and an additional six participated as competitors. The Supreme Council of Olympic Councils of Africa, representing 45 nations, has officially recognized FICS for athletic events in Africa, and recognition has been obtained from the Soviet Sports Council.

Membership of the FICS is divided into associate and full member categories. In order to become a full member a chiropractor must have five years experience in the profession and have been in practice for three years as a team doctor with an athletic or sports organization. In addition there is a complex points system to satisfy. This is based on such aspects as experience, knowledge of languages, attendance at approved symposia, contributions to sports medicine journals, and membership of national sports councils. The United States Certified Chiropractic Sports Physician diploma will provide an applicant with half of the required points. Only full members may travel abroad with teams and athletes to international events where the FICS credential is recognized.

WORLD FEDERATION OF CHIROPRACTIC

At the World Chiropractic Presidents' Summit in London in September 1987 a working party was appointed to consult with chiropractors in 49 countries before presenting a draft constitution for a body that would represent chiropractors in the international health care world. As a result a draft constitution was approved in Sydney, Australia, in October 1988 creating the World Federation of Chiropractic, and this has since been launched following ratification by each national association.

The WFC has already begun its work by representing the chiropractic profession at the World Health Organization. It serves as a forum for the discussion of common professional issues, and aims to develop a central database and library. One of its key functions is to assist in the establishment of appropriate chiropractic legislation world-wide.

The Federation is controlled by a Council of 11 chiropractic leaders elected on a regional basis. These regions are similar to those established by the WHO, namely Africa, Asia, Eastern Mediterranean, Europe, Latin America, North America, and the Pacific. Its Secretariat is established in Toronto, and Mr David Chapman-Smith, an attorney who played a key role in chiropractic's presentation before New Zealand's Commission of Inquiry, has been appointed its Chief Executive Officer. All major established health professions are represented at the WHO by such bodies, and the WFC symbolizes for chiropractic its position as a major force within today's world health care system.

Chapter 12

CHIROPRACTIC'S PLACE IN THE HEALTH CARE SYSTEM

Health is a state of complete physical, mental, and social well-being and not merely the absence of disease or infirmity. *World Health Organization Constitution* (1948)

RELATIONSHIP WITH MEDICINE

In Switzerland chiropractic has long been established as a registered profession, and this stability has allowed it to heal old wounds and develop a healthy relationship with the medical profession that has brought great benefit to patients. There is a common understanding between the two professions which makes cross-referral of patients simple, swift, and effective, in contrast to those countries where this relationship has not developed, and where patients feel unwittingly caught up in the middle of a conflict not of their making.

In Britain there is a growing dissatisfaction with the medical health service, not for its emergency cover which is amongst the best in the world, but for its management of non life-threatening illness. Not only are patients flocking to 'alternative' practitioners, but many doctors now attend weekend courses in subjects like acupuncture and manipulation. While patients realize that few doctors have any expertise in these alternative methods, they remain lost in a sea of bogus qualifications when seeking help outside the medical profession. They are often unsure of consulting their general practitioner for fear of upsetting them, and therefore tend to turn to alternative therapists on the word of a friend, neighbour, or colleague at work. Experience of the non-medical approach is therefore haphazard for many.

Qualified chiropractors have so far been denied any statutory status that would establish their training and ethical standards, and consequently the public have no way of knowing the background of a practitioner. Patients run the risk of being robbed, abused, or disillusioned as they experience 'manipulation' at the hands of unscrupulous incompetents, blatant amateurs and well-meaning but ill-trained medical practitioners.

Qualified chiropractors are fighting to lay down in Britain the standards of chiropractic training and scope of practice that are accepted internationally within the chiropractic community. In countries where these standards have been enshrined in law we are witnessing a movement towards the breaking of inter-professional antagonism, towards the cross-referral of patients, towards medical health insurance cover for chiropractic care, and towards full acceptance of chiropractic treatment for those conditions which are seen to respond so well.

This process has already begun on a very limited scale in Britain, where increasing numbers of general practitioners are referring their patients to registered members of the British Chiropractic Association. This has been helped by the government's Medical Research Council managing and partially funding a trial to compare medical and chiropractic management of back pain that should be ready for publication in 1990. A number of major private medical insurances are either designating experienced chiropractors as specialists on the recommendation of the BCA Peer Review Panel, or are providing cover to patients of BCA members. These advances into private health insurance are, however, subject to medical referral and the patient is required to seek assistance from an open-minded general practitioner before commencing treatment. Progress depends on an increasing number of free-thinking medical doctors, or on insurance companies accepting actuarial figures from overseas that demonstrate chiropractic's cost-effectiveness. Barriers to co-operation are certain to remain so long as chiropractic training and standards remain undefined in law.

In America the success of chiropractic's anti-trust suits has forced the grudging acceptance of chiropractic by the medical community. This has led to considerable co-operation between ordinary medical doctors and chiropractors, and cross referrals and the use of hospital diagnostic facilities are becoming common place.

In retaliation organized medicine is trying to turn the tables on

its old adversary by promoting manipulation by physiotherapists, and then claiming that chiropractic's opposition to their
often primitive techniques amounts in turn to anti-trust activity.
It remains to be seen how successfully this ploy will develop.

RELATIONSHIP WITHIN THE MANIPULATIVE PROFESSIONS

The relationship of chiropractors with osteopaths, physiotherapists, and the various medical and non-medical manipulators is
a very mixed one. Osteopaths have tended to regard D.D. Palmer
as the cuckoo who laid his golden chiropractic egg in the
osteopathic nest, whereas chiropractors have accused osteopaths
of using time-wasting and non-specific techniques and of allying
with orthodox medicine against them. Chiropractors and
osteopaths both regard physiotherapists as opportunists
dabbling in manipulation, poaching but not perfecting their
techniques, carrying them into hospitals to use as their own,
while physiotherapists from the safe confines of the medical
establishment look on their longer trained rivals as 'unqualified'.
Few medical manipulators have any genuine manipulative
training, yet they label the real experts in the field as 'lay
manipulators'. Chiropractors and osteopaths look on medical
manipulators as inadequate imitators of their art, all too ready to
reach for the needle and inject anti-inflammatory drugs to hide
a lack of expertise. Lay manipulators are generally regarded by all
parties as ignorant and dangerous, although very often they are
the sole remnants of the bonesetting tradition whose inspiration
set the chiropractic, osteopathic, and medical manipulative
professions on their evolutionary trail. What is highly ironic is
that few of the genuine experts in manipulative therapy are yet
eligible for health insurance cover, whilst such cover is readily
granted by insurers to a medical practitioner with no qualification in manipulation save a brass plate outside the door.

The picture of various groups squabbling over the share of the
cake is largely universal. American chiropractors look on their
osteopathic colleagues as pseudo-medics, and it is ironic that
manipulation is only optional in some osteopathic colleges
where the osteopath is taught to prescribe drugs and to perform
surgery. In Australia qualified chiropractors resent being clubbed

together under one statute with large numbers of osteopaths of questionable training who entered the state registers under a 'grandfather clause'. Whereas more than 98 per cent of chiropractors the world over share a common background, level of training, and system of mutual recognition, osteopathy ranges from a branch of allopathic medicine at one extreme to scantily trained bonesetters at the other. One of the few countries where chiropractors and osteopaths have been able to co-operate on a limited level is Great Britain. Here the British Chiropractic Association was able to lend its support to the General Council and Register of Osteopaths for their Osteopaths Bill in 1986, as this leading osteopathic body shares a common legislative goal with chiropractors.

RELATIONSHIP WITH ALTERNATIVE MEDICINE

Since its inception chiropractic has largely distanced itself from alternative medicine the world over in spite of government bodies and established medicine trying to lump all non-medical approaches together in one big pot. It may be that the more dubious reputation of some of the more questionable 'alternatives' is intended to rub off on more scientifically based chiropractic and osteopathy. In West Germany chiropractors have no legal identity other than that bestowed upon them as 'heilpraktikers' (health practitioners), and they have difficulty in establishing themselves as a specialist manipulative profession.

From the earliest roots of chiropractic history D.D. and then B.J. Palmer were critical of alternative medicine. The Straights believed most emphatically that as the subluxation was at the root of all disease only its removal would ensure a permanent cure. They accepted that diet and psychological irritants could play a part in the build up to a subluxation, but rarely went further than giving cursory advice on avoidance. On the other hand, many a Mixer incorporated naturopathy, massage, homoeopathy, herbal medicine, or acupuncture as an adjunctive therapy, and the proponents of applied kinesiology have taken on board acupuncture meridians and dietary supplementation within a chiropractic setting.

Although chiropractors in their early years chose to fight alone, in more recent years they have broken down these barriers when their continued survival has been threatened by orthodox medicine. In South Africa, when faced with total extinction, chiropractors, homoeopaths, naturopaths, osteopaths, and herbalists fought side-by-side to carve an independent place for themselves in the South African health care system.

In Britain, reflecting their early Straight philosophy, chiropractors remained aloof from alternative medicine until 1945 when the Welfare State threatened the provision of non-medical health care. Sharing as a common goal the continuation of their livelihoods they worked together as the Joint Committee of Unorthodox Practitioner Associations. When they had achieved only a limited advancement of their cause the various groups resumed their bickering and went their separate ways. A number of attempts in the 1950s, 1960s, and 1970s to bring unorthodox groups together failed to gain any momentum, until another threat appeared on the horizon. In support of alternative medicine, H.R.H. The Prince of Wales called for the orthodox medical profession to look more carefully at other forms of healing. The British Medical Association announced that its Board of Science would investigate the 'alternatives'. A cursory glance at the make-up of the investigative board and its known hard-liners gave cause for concern, and prompted a serious attempt by the more established professions to come together. At the same time the Greater London Council General Powers Bill was attempting to lump tattooists with acupuncturists, and chiropractors and osteopaths with massage parlours under a licence of premises law. Government, the media, and public bodies called for a single body for them to deal with, and after a couple of years of informal meetings the Council for Complementary and Alternative Medicine launched itself publicly at the House of Lords in February 1985 under the auspices of former Prime Minister Lord Home of the Hirsel. Chiropractic, Acupuncture, Medical Herbalism, Osteopathy, and Homoeopathy are each represented on the Council, which meets monthly to discuss and form common ground on current issues. Ethical standards for the professions were rapidly agreed, but educational needs vary so widely between them that it has not been possible to agree on common minimum standards. The Council has therefore sub-divided itself into categories, and is busy laying the path of educational accreditation for the first category, acupuncture.

A VISION FOR THE FUTURE

It would probably be unrealistic to dream that one day chiropractic, conventional, and alternative medicine will share joint responsibility for the health of the world, although from a humanitarian point of view this is the obvious answer. For a vision of the future to have any value it has to be more substantial than the stuff that dreams are made of.

It is unlikely that medicine will wish to regard chiropractic as a separate speciality for the treatment of back pain, and the dream of chiropractors for independent back-care specialist status based upon the tooth-care specialist model of dentists is unlikely to materialize. Medicine will continue to train physio-therapists in manipulation in an attempt to take over the territory occupied by chiropractic and osteopathy, although their efforts in this field are still too simplistic to risk supplanting the genuine specialists in the near future. It is unlikely that governments will be able to ignore for long the balanced judgement of independent commissions such as those of New Zealand and Sweden, and chiropractic will continue to win its legislative battles, particularly in Scandinavia and Europe where registration is long overdue. There will be attempts in some countries to bring chiropractic and osteopathy together as one profession, but historic differences are too deep and therapeutic approaches too dissimilar for this to be successful in the short term, and this ploy may be used by the medical lobby in an attempt to divide and conquer.

The continued registration of chiropractors in Europe will help to stabilize the profession, allowing it to devote more energy to research and validation of chiropractic methods, and chiro-practic colleges will become established in several European countries and in Scandinavia. Britain has already followed the Australian lead by having its chiropractic qualification accredited as a recognized degree, and this will facilitate post-graduate study and research projects with universities and hospitals. Degree status is likely to enhance chiropractic's reputation at grass-root level with most medical practitioners, and we shall see more written referrals to chiropractors, replacing the 'under the table' verbal referrals which occur frequently at present. Increased competition in the health insurance market will put pressure on the major insurers to include chiropractic cover, aided by the involvement of large employers who wish their employees to benefit from the cost-effectiveness of chiropractic care. At first this will be subject to medical referral only, and attempts to obtain cover independent of medicine will take longer to achieve. Possibly it will not occur until the British health service has adapted its structure to resemble more efficient overseas models.

In many countries there is likely to be a parallel growth and stabilization of the osteopathic professions, although they will probably lag behind in Europe on the educational and research front as few colleges are likely to achieve a degree level education in the near future. During this catching-up period it is possible that chiropractic could evolve a reputation for being of a more specialist nature than osteopathy, especially with the move towards an honours degree in chiropractic.

As osteopathy and chiropractic become more respectable there will be claims within medicine that they are able to provide these services themselves. With increasing competition in their own ranks more young doctors will embark upon short training courses in manipulation. Medicine will try to incorporate manipulative therapy into physiotherapy and orthopaedic departments within the National Health Service, and will attempt to distance itself from chiropractic and osteopathy, perhaps driving a wedge between these two professions in an attempt to keep them both beyond the pale. Continued rejection by medicine and its encroachment into manipulation are likely to reawaken interest in chiropractic and osteopathic philosophies. This will prompt chiropractors and osteopaths to turn their research efforts into validating the effects of their treatment on the autonomic nervous system pathways. As newly established professions with more research facilities open to them, it is likely that they will get nearer to explaining why manipulation is successful in so many 'organic' conditions, and criteria will be established to help select suitable cases for treatment.

Chiropractors will therefore remain on the fringes of conventional medicine, which will continue to reject them as non-medical. This scenario is not a totally negative one, for it will force chiropractors to continue their pioneering efforts into directions that conventional medicine, by its very nature, cannot follow. Yet from the safe confines of a registered profession chiropractic will be able to maintain its ethical and educational standards and will take up its place as part of the establishment in its own right.

The process of working from within a registered profession will begin with the chiropractors and osteopaths, whose success in the treatment of back pain is readily verified by research, and whose educational standards are generally far ahead of those in the alternative medicine professions. Nevertheless, the legislative, educational, and research successes of chiropractic and osteopathy are likely to be followed in time by the major branches of alternative medicine, which will experience the same encroachments from medicine into those aspects of their practice which are compatible with allopathy. Again this will drive them back to the roots of their philosophies, and those who are able to withstand this process will be able to develop a more powerful alternative to allopathy based upon sound education and research, and from within the strong bastions of an established and registered profession.

Pessimists look on the might of the massive medical lobby and preach the demise of chiropractic and alternative medicine within a century, as allopathy gobbles up those parts it can comfortably digest. Other pessimists look upon the attempts of chiropractors and osteopaths to upgrade their basic science and diagnostic studies as panderings to medicine, and foretell the absorption of both into the medical machine, as has happened to osteopathy in America. Optimists look on the squirmings of the medical profession as they try to talk their way out of massive iatrogenic disasters such as thalidomide, opren, and other catastrophic drugs. Such people foresee a public reaction against allopathic medicine and a flocking to alternative medicine. None of these pictures represents a realistic image of the next century.

Conventional medicine is here to stay, and in many dramatic ways it can demonstrate its life-saving properties as it transplants kidneys, saves leukaemic children, and renews elderly joints with metal and plastic. Nevertheless it believes inherently that disease must be fought with drugs, with the knife, and with heroic methods, and although it may pay lip-service to prevention and to the holistic approach, few medical students carry this through to the end of their training, and fewer still sustain it in practice.

The public will always need an alternative approach, whether it be provided by a registered complementary practitioner, by an unregistered alternative therapist, or by a faith healer. Whatever its professional status, practising within or outide of the law, an alternative unorthodox approach will always survive.

GLOSSARY

The following are chiropractic, medical, or general terms which may be encountered when reading about chiropractic or the conditions it treats.

Activator: a hand-held instrument used by some chiropractors to deliver a mechanically measured rapid thrust (adjustment).

Active movement: The action of moving a joint or joints without assistance.

Acute symptoms: symptoms that are severe and have reached a painfully sharp crisis.

Adjustment: the highly-controlled specific manipulation used by chiropractors.

   Indirect adjustment: adjustment of a joint using a point of contact distant to that joint.

Allopathic medicine: orthodox medical practice.

Alternative medicine: a form of medicine not generally provided in orthodox medical practice, and often rejected by it.

Angina pectoris: a heart condition characterized by sudden attacks of agonizing pain, usually in the chest or left arm, which goes after several minutes of rest.

Ankylosing spondylitis: an inflammatory condition of the spine leading progressively to a fusing together of vertebrae.

Ankylosis: a growing together or fusion of joint surfaces leading to total immobility of the joint.

Applied kinesiology: a system of analysis and treatment based on a fusion of chiropractic and acupuncture philosophy. It links the function of an organ to specific muscle groups, vertebrae, acupuncture meridians, and nerve, blood vessel and lymphatic stimulation points.

Arthritis: inflammation of a joint.

Osteoarthrosis: the commonest form of arthritis, caused by degenerative changes in a joint.

Rheumatoid arthritis: a form of arthritis related to a malfunction of the body's auto-immune system.

Spondylosis: osteoarthrosis of the spinal joints.

Atlas: the topmost vertebra of the spine, lying between the base of the skull (occiput) and the axis.

Atrophy: a wasting away of muscles, bones or other tissues.

Autonomic nervous system: *see* Nervous system.

Axis: the second vertebra of the spine that lies between the Atlas and the third cervical vertebra.

Balans furniture: Scandinavian furniture designed to allow a person to sit or work at a surface with the minimum of strain.

Basic sciences: science subjects that form the foundation of studies in the healing arts and include subjects such as anatomy, physiology, biochemistry, histology, microbiology, embryology, and pathology.

Biomechanics: study of the structural, functional and mechanical aspects of human or animal movement.

Blocks: wedge-shaped devices designed to apply a corrective therapeutic force using gravity alone.

Body mechanics: study of the human body in motion and the application of treatment to restore optimum function.

Carpal tunnel syndrome: a condition characterized by hand pain or pins and needles which may involve symptoms higher in the arm. It is due to swelling within the wrist pressurizing a nerve.

Case History: a patient's medical history, including that of the presenting complaint.

Central Nervous System: *see* Nervous system.

Cervical spine: the uppermost region of the spine that includes the seven vertebrae of the neck. The occiput lies above and the thoracic spine below.

Chiropractic: an independent branch of medicine specializing in mechanical disorders of the joints, particularly those of the spine, and their effects upon the nervous system. Treatment is mainly by specific manipulation (adjustment) of joints and soft tissues.

Chronic symptoms: symptoms which are deep-seated and long-lasting.

Coccyx: triangular shaped tail bone consisting of 3–5 fused rudimentary vertebrae. It is attached to the sacrum above and terminates the vertebral column below. Pain in the coccyx is known as coccydynia.

Compensation: secondary changes which occur in the body in response to a primary condition.

Complementary medicine: a form of medicine which supplies a deficiency in conventional medical practice.

Connective tissues: those fibrous and membranous tissues which with cartilage, bone and certain cells fulfil a structural role, and which with other cells provide a defensive role against disease.

Contraindication: a factor which prohibits, or renders undesirable, certain forms of treatment.

Cranial: pertaining to the skull. Cranial adjustment involves manually influencing the minute movements of the skull which accompany breathing.

Cranial nerve: *see* Nerve.

Creep effect: the deformative changes which occur in soft tissues in response to sustained bending or loading.

Degenerative joint disease: osteoarthrosis. *See* Arthritis.

Diagnosis: the identification of a disease from its signs and symptoms.

Disc: a disc of fibrocartilage found in certain joints. Intervertebral discs form the chief bonds of connexion between adjacent vertebral bodies from the axis to the sacrum and function primarily for weight bearing.

Herniated or prolapsed disc: protrusion of the soft nucleus of an intervertebral disc through its hard fibrous annular lining, where it may induce irritation of a spinal nerve root.

Slipped disc: a misnomer applied to many spinal conditions that may benefit from chiropractic treatment, the usual being a bulge in the disc that may irritate a spinal nerve root.

Drop technique: a chiropractic technique which uses a sectional drop treatment table. The section is set at an appropriate tension so that it falls away about an inch when the chiropractic thrust is delivered. The resultant momentum is designed to augment the affects of the adjustment.

Eclectic medicine: a broad system of medicine based upon the selection and reconciliation of various principles belonging to different schools of thought. Often used as an antonym to allopathic medicine.

Elastic barrier of resistance: the resistance felt at the limit of a joint's range of passive movement. With a correctly applied adjustment the joint is carried painlessly beyond the barrier but within the joint's anatomical range of movement, thereby increasing its mobility.

Endocrine system: that system of tissues and organs which gives rise to internal hormonal secretions.

Facet joint: one of a pair of small vertebral joints which lie posterior to the intervertebral disc. Facet (posterior) joints are responsible for conducting the fine guiding movements of vertebrae but not for weight bearing. Incorrect posture or strains commonly overload the facets, which are more pain sensitive than intervertebral discs, and they provide the most frequent source of spinal pain.

Fascia: a sheet of membranous tissue investing the softer more delicate organs.

Femoral nerve: one of the major nerves which passes down the thigh and leads from the lumbar spine. Irritation of its nerve root (femoral neuralgia) can induce pain or pins and needles down the front of the thigh.

Fibrositis: inflammatory changes to white fibrous tissue, especially to those of muscle linings or fascia. Often used as a loose term to describe painful shoulder muscles.

Fibrous tissue: membranous elastic, non-elastic or net-like connective tissues, such as those which line the muscles or organs, which are composed of multiple fibres.

Fight or flight response: the primitive reactions which occur posturally and within the body in response to a threatening situation.

Fixation: the partial or full restriction of a joint within its normal range of movement. A hypomobile joint.

Foramen: a natural opening in a bone which carries blood vessels and/or nerves.

Intervertebral foramen: one of a pair of openings between two adjacent vertebrae which transmits spinal nerves and blood vessels to and from the spinal cord.

Frozen shoulder: *see* Retractile capsulitis.

Functional: relating to the performance of organs, muscles, joints, or other structures but not to their physical structure.

Heel lift: a thin wedge-shaped appliance, usually of cork, which is slipped into the shoe to raise the heel.

Hole in one: a technique developed by B.J. Palmer based on the premise that specific adjustment of the atlas or axis is sufficient to restore full and healthy function of the body and nervous system. Also known as Specific (or Palmer) Upper Cervical Technique.

Homoeostasis: that state of equilibrium which maintains the interrelating systems and functions of the healthy body.

Hypermobility: a state of excessive mobility within a joint.

Hypomobility: a state of insufficient mobility within a joint.

Impingement: encroachment upon a nerve or other structure causing it to be moved away from its natural position.

Indirect adjustment: *see* Adjustment.

Innate intelligence: the inborn intelligence within every individual that is responsible for maintaining and co-ordinating bodily function and health.

Instability: that state of joint malfunction which allows it to move excessively (hypermobility), usually incurring inflammation and pain.

Intervertebral disc: *see* Disc.

Isometric exercise: exercise designed to build up muscle strength without muscle growth by holding the muscle in a steady state of resisted contraction, usually for about five seconds per contraction.

Isotonic exercise: exercise designed to build up muscle strength and bulk by repeated movement, lengthening and shortening the muscle under tension.

Kyphosis: an exaggerated backward curvature of the thoracic spine.

Ligament: a band of fibrous tissue which binds bones together or holds tendons, muscles or organs in place.

Locomotor system: that system which directs the physical movement of the body, and includes muscles, tendons, ligaments, joints and bones.

Lordosis: an exaggerated forward curvature of the lumbar or cervical spine.

Lumbago: a loose term used to describe backache in the lumbar region of the spine.

Lumbar spine: the low back region of the spine whose five vertebrae lie above the sacrum and below the thoracic spine.

Lymphatic fluids: the fluids (lymph) which bathe and nourish tissues of the body and collect waste or invasive materials for processing.

Manipulation: therapeutic application of a manual force.

Mental impulse: impulses from the brain directing tissue and cell function through the nervous system.

Meric system: treatment of visceral conditions by adjusting vertebrae at their neuromeric levels. The neuromeric level is that part of a nerve's pathway between an organ and its spinal or autonomic nerve outlet where it passes through or near to a vertebral joint.

Migraine: hemicranial pain. A condition characterized by recurrent one sided, frontal, or temporal headaches accompanied by visual disturbances, nausea, vomiting, or light sensitivity.

Mobilization: a manoeuvre, less specific than an adjustment, designed to increase the range of movement of a structure.

Motion palpation: *see* Palpation.

Motor pathway: the path taken by a nerve whose function is to carry excitatory impulses from the central nervous system to induce movement of a muscle or other organ. *See* Nerve, Nervous system.

Motor unit: *see* Vertebral motor unit.

Musculo-skeletal system: that system pertaining to the inter-relationship of muscles and bones. *See* Locomotor system.

Nerve: a bundle of fibres which carries electrical impulses from one part of the nervous system to another.

Cranial nerve: one of twelve pairs of peripheral nerves arising directly from the brain.

Motor nerve: a nerve which carries impulses from the central nervous system to effect an action elsewhere.

Peripheral nerve: a cranial or spinal nerve.

Sensory nerve: a nerve which conveys sensation to the central nervous system.

Somatic nerve: a sensory or motor nerve which supplies the framework of the body.

Spinal nerve: one of the 31 pairs of peripheral nerves attached to the spinal cord.

Nerve root: that part of a peripheral nerve where it attaches to the central nervous system. Neuralgia usually derives from nerve root irritation due to its close proximity to vertebral structures.

Nervous system: the electrical system which governs the creation, co-ordination, and passage of impulses from one structure to another.

Autonomic nervous system: that part of the nervous system which functions independently of the will, and is subdivided into sympathetic and parasympathetic elements.

Central nervous system: that part of the nervous system composed of the brain and spinal cord which governs and co-ordinates its function.

Parasympathetic nervous system: that division of the autonomic nervous system arising from the cranial nerves and the sacral nerves (spinal nerves of the sacrum).

Peripheral nervous system: that part of the nervous system composed of the spinal and cranial nerves.

Sympathetic nervous system: the larger division of the autonomic nervous system which arises from the thoracic and lumbar spinal nerves.

Neuralgia: pain in the distribution or course of a nerve.

Neurocalometer (NCM): an instrument designed to detect heat differences either side of a vertebra.

Neuromuscular technique: a form of treatment based upon the stimulation or elimination of trigger points.

Neuro-musculo-skeletal system: the system of nervous, muscular and skeletal structures which governs and co-ordinates locomotor activity.

Nimmo receptor tonus method: a method of chiropractic treatment which complements adjustment with the application of pressure upon a trigger point.

Non-force technique: a method of treatment which avoids the application of a direct mobilizing thrust to a joint.

Occiput: the cranial bone which lies at the back of the head and articulates with the atlas.

Organic: relating to the organs (viscera) of the body.

Orthopaedic: relating to disorders of the locomotor system.

Osteoarthrosis: *see* Arthritis.

Osteomalacia: softening of the bone.

Osteophyte: an abnormal outgrowth of dense bone, usually part of the degenerative process of a joint.

Painful arc: that part within a joint's normal range of movement which is accompanied by pain on movement.

Palpation: examination with the hand.

Motion palpation: manual examination of a structure during movement to assess its functional capacity.

Static palpation: manual examination of a structure at rest to assess its functional capacity.

Palpitation: a sensation of fluttering usually applied to the awareness of an unduly rapid or irregular heart beat.

Paraspinal: related to structures situated alongside the spine.

Passive movement: the action of moving a resting joint using another unrelated part of the body, or movement of that joint by another person.

Pelvis: the basin-like structure situated at the base of the trunk and formed by two hip bones (each composed of an ileum and ischium fused together), the sacrum, and the coccyx, and their associated ligaments. The movable vertebrae arise from the sacrum, and the pelvis as a whole transmits weight from the trunk to the legs.

Physical examination: examination of the body.

Piriformis muscle: one of the hip muscles, often unduly contracted in certain low back conditions.

Posterior gravity line: a common postural condition whereby the lower lumbar curve is increased, stressing postural muscles, ligaments, and facet joints.

Posterior joint: *see* Facet joint.

Posture: the stance and carriage of the bodily frame.

Postural distortion: a departure from the normal postural status of the healthy human frame.

Prone: lying face downwards.

Psoas muscle: one of the hip muscles which, as the ilio-psoas, connects to the upper lumbar vertebrae and may be implicated in a number of spinal or postural conditions.

Radiculitis: irritation of a nerve root usually inducing referred pain.

Range of movement: the degree of movement that can be elicited from a joint.

Reaction: a symptom which appears as a result of treatment.

Adverse reaction: detrimental symptoms arising from an incorrect therapeutic approach.

Normal reaction: symptoms which may sometimes arise after treatment either from the process of retracing or from the resuscitation of tissues that have atrophied from lack of use. Such reactions are normally short-lived.

Referred pain: pain felt in a location distant from the involved site.

Reflex: the involuntary action of transferring an ingoing stimulus into an outgoing impulse through the mediation of the central nervous system.

Pathological reflex: the process whereby irritation of a structure initiates a harmful response in tissues which lie at the end of its associated reflex arc. *See* Reflex arc.

Somato-autonomic reflex: a reflex whereby an impulse originating in the soma (body) is converted to a secondary action through the autonomic nervous system, for example, a vertebral disorder leading to migraine. *See Somato-visceral reflex.*

Somato-somatic reflex: a reflex whereby an impulse originating in the soma (body) is converted to an action elsewhere in the soma, for example, a cervical joint disorder inducing shoulder muscle contraction and pain.

Somato-visceral reflex: a reflex whereby an impulse originating in the soma (body) is converted to an action in the viscera (organs), for example, a lumbar joint disorder inducing painful menstruation or constipation.

Viscero-somatic reflex: a reflex whereby an impulse originating in an organ is converted to an action in the soma (body), for example, gall bladder disease inducing pain and contraction in the right shoulder.

Viscero-visceral reflex: a reflex whereby an impulse originating in an organ is converted to an action in another organ, for example, a heart attack inducing nausea or vomiting.

Reflex arc: the neurological pathway through which an impulse passes into the central nervous system and out again to effect a response.

Reflex test: functional assessment of a reflex arc by applying a stimulating force, as in tapping one of the deep tendons with a rubber tipped reflex hammer. One common example, the knee tap test, assesses the reflex pathway via the fourth lumbar nerve to the spinal cord and back to the quadriceps muscle, which then momentarily contracts.

Restriction: full or partial limitation of normal joint movement. Fixation, hypomobility.

Retracing: the process whereby correction of a condition is accompanied by the reappearance of symptoms which had been present when the condition was forming but which had subsequently been masked. Such reactions are normally short-lived.

Retractile capsulitis: inflammatory changes which occur to the fibrous sheath surrounding a joint, and which restrict its movement. Often applied to the 'frozen shoulder', when no movement is possible beyond that permitted by the muscular attachments at the back of the shoulder blade.

Rheumatism: a condition marked by sharp pain and swelling in joints and their associated muscles. Often used as a loose term to describe chronic aching muscles.

Rheumatoid arthritis: *see* Arthritis.

Sacro-iliac joint: one of a pair of fibrous weight-bearing joints lying between the sacrum and ileum. Any restriction of its small degree of movement can induce compensatory stress to the lower lumbar spine. If excessively mobile it can become acutely inflamed, usually after childbirth.

Sacro-occipital technique (SOT): a system of analysis and treatment based on a fusion of chiropractic philosophy with Sutherland's cranial osteopathy. It holds that the process of respiration (breathing) is accompanied by counterbalancing cranial and sacral movements, and that malfunction of this mechanism inhibits cerebrospinal fluid flow and initiates organic disorders. Treatment is aimed at restoring the counterbalance of cranium and sacrum.

Sacrum: a large triangular bone composed of five fused sacral vertebrae inserted in a wedge-like manner between the two hip bones (ilia). Forming the back of the pelvis, it articulates above with the lumbar spine and below with the coccyx.

Sciatica: intense referred pain felt along the distribution of the sciatic nerve, especially at the back of the thigh. As the largest nerve in the body, the sciatic nerve leaves the spinal cord through the lower lumbar vertebrae and upper sacrum, passes through the pelvis, supplies the back of the thigh, and leads to nerves of the leg, foot and toes.

Scoliosis: an abnormal sideways curve or series of curves in the spinal column.

Sensory pathway: the anatomical pathway of a sensory nerve, whose function is to carry sensation to the central nervous system. *See* Nerve, Nervous system.

Short leg: an anatomical, pathological or functional deficiency of leg length on one side.

Functional short leg: the appearance of a short leg caused by muscular or postural deficiencies. Correction of the deficiency restores normal leg length.

Slipped disc: *see* Disc.

Soft tissues: those tissues of the body which yield to pressure, such as muscles, ligaments, tendons, and fibrous tissues. Soft tissue treatments include massage, pressure, mobilization, friction, goading and stretching of the tissues.

Somatic: pertaining to the physical body (soma).
Somatic dysfunction: impaired function of the somatic system.
Somatic nervous system: *see* Nervous system.
Somatic reflex: *see* Reflex.
Somatic system: that system composed of skeletal, joint, muscular, fibrous tissue, and related blood vessel, lymphatic, and neurological elements.

Specific (Palmer) upper cervical technique: *see* Hole in one.

Spinal column: *see* Vertebral column.

Spinal cord: that part of the central nervous system leaving the brainstem and passing down through the vertebral column to give rise to the spinal nerves.

Spinal mechanics: study of the structural, functional, and mechanical aspects of spinal movement.

Spinous process: the most readily palpable part of a vertebra, felt in the midline as a hard nodular projection. Commonly referred to as a vertebral 'spine'.

Spondylitis: inflammation of a spinal joint that may lead to spondylosis. *See* Arthritis.

Spondylolisthesis: forward displacement of a vertebra on the one below, usually occurring when the fifth lumbar vertebra slides forward on the sacrum.

Sprain: joint injury involving rupture of some, but not all, of the fibres of a supporting ligament.

Strain: overstretching and tearing of some of the fibres of a muscle or other connective tissue.

Subluxation: a term used by chiropractors to describe an abnormality of vertebral function. It is occasionally applied to non spinal joints.

Primary or major subluxation: a subluxation which, by its very nature, induces a secondary subluxation elsewhere. Adjustment is often directed to a primary subluxation first in an attempt to spontaneously eliminate secondary subluxations.

Secondary subluxation: a subluxation which has occurred as a direct result of and as a compensation for a primary subluxation elsewhere.

Supine: lying face upwards.

System: a group of organs which function in a complex organized manner for a specialized purpose. Examples are the circulatory, digestive, endocrine, locomotor (musculo-skeletal), nervous, reproductive, respiratory, and urinary systems.

Technique: a physical procedure used to treat patients.

Tendon: a tough fibrous cord which anchors muscle to its bony attachments.

Thompson terminal point technique: a form of chiropractic analysis based on the premise that subluxation patterns result from patterns of muscle contracture and that certain leg length tests reveal these patterns. Adjustment is on a sectional drop table. *See* Drop technique.

Thoracic spine: that region of the spine whose twelve vertebrae provide attachment for the twelve sets of ribs which form the thorax. It lies below the cervical and above the lumbar regions of the spine.

Thrust: the controlled sudden directional force or drive which accompanies a chiropractic adjustment.

Tinnitus: a condition marked by continuous ringing in the ear.

Toggle recoil: a chiropractic adjustment marked by a rapid thrust followed by a recoiling away of the operator's hands.

Tone or Tonus:
Of a muscle: the basic tension of a muscle at rest. In skeletal muscle it aids the maintenance of posture.

Of a nerve: the basic impulses discharged along a nerve at rest.

Torticollis: a spasmodic contraction of neck muscles which draws the head to one side. Wry neck.

Trigger point: a small nodule of contracted and irritable tissue that, when compressed, is locally tender and may give rise to referred pain or autonomic symptoms. Therapeutic pressure may eliminate the reflex arc that is associated with it, breaking related symptoms and at times erasing the primary stimulus.

Unstable joint: *see* Instability.

Vertebra: one of the 32–34 bones that form the backbone (vertebral column).

Vertebral column: the backbone, composed of 7 cervical (neck), 12 thoracic (middle and upper back), 5 lumbar (lower back), 5 sacral (pelvis), and 3–5 coccygeal (tailbone) vertebral segments.

Vertebral motor unit: those elements linking two adjacent vertebrae and consisting of the intervertebral disc, facet (posterior) joints, ligaments, muscles, and associated nerves, blood vessels, lymphatics, and connective tissues.

Vertigo: a sensation of revolving within the head (giddiness, dizziness) accompanied by loss of balance. Often associated with Meniere's disease or cervical spondylosis.

Viscera: the organs of the body.

FURTHER READING

For those of you who wish to delve further into chiropractic, the following headings contain useful references.

GENERAL READING ON CHIROPRACTIC

Dintenfass, J., *Chiropractic: A Modern Way to Health*, (Pyramid, New York, 1970).

Fraser, John Lloyd, *The Medicine Men – A Guide to Natural Medicine*, pp. 65–89. (Eyre Methuen, London, 1981).

Fulder, Stephen, *The Handbook of Complementary Medicine*, pp. 151–158 (Oxford University Press, 2nd edition, 1988).

Moore, Susan, *Chiropractic*, (Mcdonald Optima, London, 1988).

Moore, Susan, 'Chiropractic Therapy', in Mills, Simon, *Alternatives in Healing*, pp. 16–23. (Macmillan, London, 1988).

Moore, Susan, *New Ways to Health – a Guide to Chiropractic* (Hamlyn, London, 1989).

Scofield, Arthur G., *Chiropractice*, (Thorsons, Wellingborough, 1977).

Sportelli, Louis, *Introduction to Chiropractic – A Natural Method of Health Care*, (Sportelli, Palmerton, USA, 8th edition 1986).

CHIROPRACTIC HISTORY

Bach, Marcus, *The Chiropractic Story*, (Si-Nel Publishing, Georgia, USA, 1986).

Gautvig, M. and Hviid, A. *Chiropractic in Denmark*, (Danish Pro-Chiropractic Association, 1975).

Gibbons, Russell W., 'The Evolution of Chiropractic: Medical and Social Protest in America', in Haldeman, Scott, *Modern Developments in the Principles and Practice of Chiropractic*, pp. 3–14, (Appleton-Century-Crofts, New York, USA, 1980).

Gielow, Vern, *Old Dad Chiro – A Biography of D.D. Palmer Founder of Chiropractic*, (Bawden Bros, Davenport, Iowa, USA, 1981).

Maynard, J.E., *Healing Hands: The Story of The Palmer Family, Discoverers and Developers of Chiropractic*, (Jonorm, Mobile, USA, 1977).

Palmer, David D., *Three Generations: A Brief History of Chiropractic*, (Palmer College of Chiropractic, Davenport, Iowa, USA, 1967).

HISTORY OF MANIPULATION

Bennett, G.M., *The Art of the Bonesetter*, (Murby, London, 1884; republished by Tamor Pierston, Isleworth, 1981).

Lomax, E., 'Manipulative Therapy: A Historical Perspective from Ancient Times to the Modern Era', in Goldstein, M., *The Research Status of Spinal Manipulative Therapy*, pp. 11–17, *NINCDS Monograph 15*, (Dept Health, Education & Welfare, Washington, DC, USA, 1975).

Schiotz, E. and Cyriax, J., *Manipulation Past and Present*, (Heinemann, London, 1975).

CHIROPRACTIC PRINCIPLES AND THEORIES

Haldeman, Scott, *Modern Developments in the Principles and*

Practice of Chiropractic, (Appleton-Century-Crofts, New York, USA, 1980).

Homewood, A.E., *The Neurodynamics of the Vertebral Subluxation*, (Privately published, Thornhill, Ontario, Canada, 1962).

Janse, J. *Principles and Practice of Chiropractic – An Anthology*, Edited Hildebrandt, R.W., (National College of Chiropractic, Lombard, Illinois, USA, 1976).

Leach, Robert A., *The Chiropractic Theories – A Synopsis of Scientific Research*, (Revised Edition, Williams and Wilkins, Baltimore, London, Los Angeles, Sydney, 1986).

SOCIOLOGICAL AND ECONOMIC ASPECTS OF CHIROPRACTIC

Breen, A.C., 'Chiropractors and the Treatment of Back Pain', *Rheumatology and Rehabilitation*, Vol. 16, No. 1, pp. 46–53, (February 1977).

Dillon, J.L., 'Health Economics and Chiropractic', *Annals Swiss Chiropractic Association*. Vol. 7, pp. 7–17. (1981).

Kelner, M., Hall, O., & Coulter, I., *Chiropractors – Do They Help? – A Study of their Education and Practice*, (Abridged Edition, Fitzhenry & Whiteside, Markham, Canada, 1986).

Wardwell, Walter I., 'Chiropractors: Challengers of Medical Domination', in Roth, J.A., *Research in the Sociology of Health Care: Changing Structures of Health Service Occupations*, Vol. 3 (JAI Press, Greenwich, Connecticut, USA, 1982).

Wardwell, Walter I., 'The Present and Future Role of the Chiropractor', in Haldeman, Scott, *Modern Developments in the Principles and Practice of Chiropractic*, (Appleton-Century-Crofts, New York, USA, 1980).

GOVERNMENT INQUIRIES

Australia: 'Chiropractic', Chapter 10 in *Medicare Benefits Review Committee, Second Report*. (Commonwealth Government Printer, Canberra, 1986).

New Zealand: 'Chiropractic in New Zealand' – *Report of the Commission of Inquiry*, (The Government Printer, Wellington, 1979).

South Africa: Steenekamp, C.S., *South Africans' Experience of Chiropractic and Homeopathy*, (Human Sciences Research Council, Pretoria, 1985).

Sweden: 'Legitimization for Vissa Kiropraktorer', *Report of Commission on Alternative Medicine*, (Social Departementete, Stockholm, English Summary, SOU 1987:12).

CHIROPRACTIC RESEARCH

Breen, A., 'Chiropractors and the Treatment of Back Pain', *Rheumatology and Rehabilitation*, Vol. 16, No. 1, pp. 46–53. (1977).

Chapman-Smith, David, *The Chiropractic Report*. P.O. Box 244, Station S, Toronto, Ontario M5M 4L7, Canada. (Published bimonthly from Nov. 1986).

Kirkaldy-Willis, W.H. and Cassidy, J.D. 'Spinal Treatment in the Treatment of Low Back Pain', *Canadian Family Physician* 31:535–540. (1985).

CHIROPRACTIC AND MEDICINE

Getzendanner, J. Wilk *et al*. vs. American Medical Association *et al*. *US District Court (Northern District of Illinois Eastern Division) No. 76 C 3777*. (Judgement dated 27 August 1987).

Motion Palpation Institute, 'Guilty of Conspiring to Destroy the Profession of Chiropractic', (MPI, Huntington Beach, California, USA, 1987).

Weiant, C.W. and Goldschmidt, S., *Medicine and Chiropractic*, (Augustin, Gluckstadt, New York, USA, 1966).

Wilk, Chester A., *Chiropractic Speaks Out*. (Wilk Publishing, Illinois, USA, 1983).

CHIROPRACTIC FROM AN INTERNATIONAL VIEWPOINT

Chapman-Smith, David, *The Chiropractic Report*. P.O. Box 244, Station S, Toronto, Ontario M5M 4L7, Canada. (Published bimonthly from Nov. 1986).

Foundation for the Advancement of Chiropractic Tenets and Science, *FACTS Bulletin – A Study of Chiropractic Worldwide*, (FACTS & International Chiropractors Association, Washington, DC. vol. 3, 1990).

USEFUL ADDRESSES

This appendix should be of use to those of you who are seeking treatment by a qualified chiropractor or who wish to take up chiropractic as a career. If you would like to know how you can help to support the advancement of chiropractic you will find the addresses of chiropractic support groups listed, and they are all eager to increase their membership so that they can represent the interests of patients more effectively.

For ease of reference you will find geographical sections, with subheadings listing the various national or international professional, patient and educational organizations. Telephone numbers have been included where possible. Most of these organizations will be happy to provide information if you are researching into aspects of chiropractic.

If you are unable to obtain details of chiropractors in countries with no national association, the *Facts Bulletin*, published jointly by FACTS and the International Chiropractors' Association (ICA), lists a number of contact names and telephone numbers. Copies of the bulletin can be ordered by writing to the ICA. (See subsection: Chiropractic in the United States.)

CHIROPRACTIC IN GREAT BRITAIN

Professional: British Chiropractic Association, 10 Greycoat Place, London SW1P 1SB. Telephone 071 222 8866. The BCA publishes a register of qualified chiropractors twice a year, a quarterly newsletter, and a periodic booklet, the *British Chiropractic Handbook*.

Patients: Chiropractic Advancement Association, 56 Barnes

Crescent, Wimbourne, Dorset BH21 2AZ. Telephone 0225 776052. The CAA publishes a quarterly newsletter for patients and others who wish to keep abreast of news at home or abroad, and there are useful articles on how to take care of your spine.

Education: Anglo-European College of Chiropractic, 13–15 Parkwood Road, Boscombe, Bournemouth, Dorset BH5 2DF. Telephone 0202 431021. A prospectus for the BSc Chiropractic degree course at AECC can be obtained by writing to the Registrar.

CHIROPRACTIC IN THE REST OF EUROPE

Professional: European Chiropractors' Union, H. Mandrup-Andersen D.C., Hon. Secretary, Ahlgade 3, 4300 Holbaek, Denmark. Telephone (45) 3-431192. The ECU publishes an annual directory of European chiropractors, listed under each constituent national association. Its professional journal, the *European Journal of Chiropractic*, is published in English by Blackwell Scientific Publications.

Patients: European Federation of Pro Chiropractic Associations, Miss T. van der Geld, Honorary Secretary, Lange Heul 59, 14033 N.E. Bussum, 12159 Netherlands. The Secretary will supply details of all patient support groups in Europe.

Education: Council on Chiropractic Education (Europe), A. Kilvaer DC, Secretary, Nansetgt. 23, N-3250 Larvik, Norway. Telephone (47) 34-83850.

CHIROPRACTIC IN AFRICA

Professional: Chiropractic Association of South Africa, 701 Poynton House, Gardiner Street, Durban 4001, Natal. Telephone (27) (31) 304-4200.

Chiropractors' Association of Zimbabwe, Medical Centre, 52 Barnes Avenue, Harare.

CHIROPRACTIC IN AUSTRALIA AND NEW ZEALAND

Professional: Australian Chiropractors' Association, Federal Secretariat, 459 Great Western Highway, Faulconbridge, New South Wales 2776. Telephone (61) (47) 515644.

United Chiropractors' Association of Australasia, P.O. Box 48, Auburn, NSW 2144. Tel (61) 2-646-2613.

New Zealand Chiropractors' Association, Ronald Sim, DC. President, P.O. Box 2858, Wellington. Telephone (64) 4-721716.

Education: Australasian Council on Chiropractic Education, Dr Stephen Bardsley, Chairman, 941 Nepean Highway, Mornington, Victoria, 3931. Telephone (61) (59) 75-3546.

CHIROPRACTIC IN CANADA

Professional: Canadian Chiropractic Association, J.L. Watkins DC, Executive Director, 1396 Eglinton Avenue West, Toronto, Ontario M6C 2E4. Telephone (1) (416) 781-5656.

Education: The Council on Chiropractic Education (Canada), Dr M.P. Henderson, President, 1494 Islington Avenue, Islington, M9A 3L5. Telephone (1) (416) 231-9502.

CHIROPRACTIC IN THE EASTERN MEDITERRANEAN

Professional: Cyprus Chiropractic Association, 11 Rodou Street, Suite 302, Nicosia 138. Telephone (357) 2-475558.

Israel Chiropractic Association, Caspi Street 20, Jerusalem. Telephone (972) 2-717464.

CHIROPRACTIC IN THE FAR EAST

Professional: Hong Kong Chiropractors' Association, Bruce S. Vaughan DC, President, 1001–2 Wing on Central Blvd., 26 Des Voeux Rd.C, Hong Kong. Telephone (852) (5) 227998.

Japanese Chiropractic Association, 3-9 3-Chome, Kita-Aoyama, Minato-Ku, Tokyo 107. Telephone (81) (3) 401-2713.

Japanese Chiropractic Doctors Association, 2621 Noborito Tama-Ku, Kawasaki. Telephone (81) (44) 933-9547.

CHIROPRACTIC IN THE UNITED STATES

Professional: American Chiropractic Association, 1701 Clarendon Blvd., Arlington, VA 22209. Telephone (1) (703) 276-8800.

International Chiropractors Association, 1110 N. Glebe Road, Suite 1000, Arlington, VA 22201. Telephone (1) (703) 528-5000.

Education: The US Council on Chiropractic Education, Dr E. Maylon Drake, President, 4401 Westown Parkway, Suite 120, West Des Moines, Iowa 50265. Telephone (1) (515) 226-9001.

INTERNATIONAL AGENCIES

Federation Internationale de Chiropractique Sportive, Stephen J. Press DC, President, 291 South Van Brunt Street, Englewood, NJ 07631, USA. Telephone (1) (201) 569-1444.

World Federation of Chiropractic, Mr David Chapman-Smith, Secretary General, P.O.Box 244, Station S, Toronto, Ontario, Canada, M5M 4L7. Telephone (1) (416) 484-9978.

Geneva address:- World Federation of Chiropractic, Case Postale 73, 1211 Geneva 16, Switzerland.

INDEX